ORGANIC FARMING AND FOOD PRODUCTION

Edited by **Petr Konvalina**

Organic Farming and Food Production
http://dx.doi.org/10.5772/45848
Edited by Petr Konvalina

Contributors

Marcelo De Andrade Ferreira, Stela Urbano, Rubem Rocha Filho, Cleber Costa, Safira Valença Bispo, Mehdi Zahaf, Leila Hamzaoui Essoussi, Karmen Pažek, Crtomir Rozman, David Frank Kings, Petr Konvalina, Albert Sundrum, Costel Samuil, Vasile Vintu, Ewa Rembiałkowska

Published by InTech

Janeza Trdine 9, 51000 Rijeka, Croatia

Publishing Process Manager Ana Pantar
Technical Editor InTech DTP team
Cover InTech Design team

Additional hard copies can be obtained from orders@intechopen.com

Organic Farming and Food Production, Edited by Petr Konvalina
p. cm.
ISBN 978-953-51-0842-9

For EU product safety concerns:
IN TECH d.o.o., Prolaz Marije Krucifikse Kozulić 3, 51000 Rijeka, Croatia,
info@intechopen.com or visit our website at intechopen.com.

Meet the editor

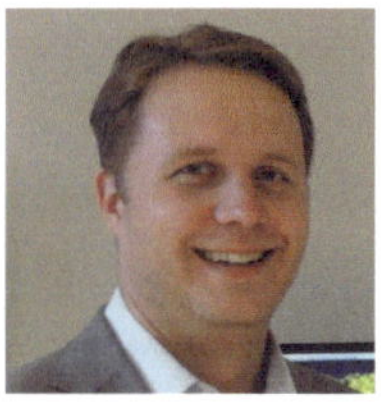

Dr. Petr Konvalina is the vice-dean for external relations at the Faculty of Agriculture, University of South Bohemia in České Budějovice, Czech Republic. He is an Associate professor in plant production. He is oriented towards organic plant production, wheat growing, organic plant breeding and organic food processing. On these topics he has published more than 100 reviewed scientific papers. The papers are mostly focused on the possibilities of practical use of genetic resources of wheat (emmer, einkorn, spelt) in organic farming. Dr. Konvalina has been involved in many national and international research and educational projects related to organic plant production.

Contents

Preface

Organic farming is a modern way of agriculture management, not using any chemical treatments which have negative effects on the environment, human health or animal health. It produces organic foodstuffs, and at the same time enhances the living conditions of animals. It contributes to environmental protection and helps biodiversity to increase. Organic farming does not mean going 'back' to traditional (old) methods of farming. Many of the farming methods used in the past are still useful today. Organic farming takes the best of these and combines them with modern scientific knowledge. Organic farmers do not let their farms to be taken over by nature; they use all their knowledge, as well as various techniques and materials available to them, in order to work with nature. In this way the farmer creates a healthy balance between nature and farming, where crops and animals can grow and thrive. To be a successful organic farmer, the farmer must not see every insect as a pest, every weed plant as out of place, nor find the solution to every problem in an artificial chemical spray. The aim is not to eradicate all pests and weeds, but to keep them down to an acceptable level and make the most of the benefits that they may provide.

The future development of organic food is never easy to predict. That is what makes it such a fascinating subject to study. At present, the sales of organic food are going through a trough and the organic industry is consolidating as it learns how to operate in a new environment. The big boom in the key markets for organic products; North America, the European Union and Japan, is faltering and the domestic purchasing power of many people is increasingly constrained (Reed, 2012). Simultaneously, organic agriculture, under the name of agro-ecology, is increasingly being presented as an answer to producing food sustainably, and improving the livelihood of farmers in the global south. A recent report from the United Nations Special Rapporteur on the Right to Food, Olivier De Schutter, which recommends the global adoption of agro-ecology, is built on the sustained effort of academic researchers to demonstrate, through high quality research, the potential of organic agriculture (De Schutter, 2011).

The book contains 8 chapters written by acknowledged experts, providing comprehesive information on all aspects of organic farming and food production. The book is divided into three parts: Organic farming, Organic food quality and sustainability and Alternative feed. In the book there are chapters oriented towards organic farming and environmental aspects, problematic organic seed production, economic optimalization of organic farming, quality and distribution of organic products, etc. Researchers, teachers and students in the agricultural field in particular will find this book to be of immense use.

The goal was to write a book where as many different existing studies as possible could be presented in a single volume, making it easy for the reader to compare methods, results and conclusions. As a result, studies from countries such as Romania, Poland, The Czech Republic, Mexico, Slovenia, Finland, etc. have been compiled into one book. I believe that the opportunity to compare results and conclusions from different countries and continents will create a new perspective in organic farming and food production. Finally, I would like to thank the contributing authors and the staff at InTech for their efforts and cooperation during the preparation of this publication. I hope that our book will help researchers and students all over the world to attain new and interesting results in the field of organic farming and food production.

Ing. Petr Konvalina, Ph.D.
Faculty of Agriculture
University of South Bohemia in České Budějovice
České Budějovice
Czech Republic

Section 1

Organic Farming

Chapter 1

Environmental Impact and Yield of Permanent Grasslands: An Example of Romania

Samuil Costel and Vintu Vasile

Additional information is available at the end of the chapter

http://dx.doi.org/10.5772/52006

1. Introduction

Organic farming is both a philosophy and a system of agricultural production. Its roots are to be found in certain values that closely reflect the ecological and social realities. Organic agriculture is a production method that takes into account the traditional knowledge of farmers and integrates the scientific progress in all agricultural disciplines, answering the social concerns of the environment and providing high quality products to consumers. The principles underpinning organic farming are universal, but the techniques used are adapted to the climatic conditions, resources and local traditions.

In other words, organic agriculture deals with the systematic study of material and functional structures of agricultural systems and the design of agro-ecosystem management capable to ensure the human needs for food, clothing and housing, for a long period of time, without diminishing the ecological, economic and social potential.

Organic farming methods to obtain food by means of culture that protect the environment and exclude the use of pesticides and synthetic fertilizers. No doubt that organic farming can also be defined as the activity of assembling the theoretical knowledge about nature and agriculture in sustainable technological systems based on material, energy and information resources of the agricultural systems. Also, organic farming is based on wisdom and as such, it involves detailed knowledge of land, living things and other economic and social realities, as well as intuition, moderation in choosing and implementing measures in practice.

Being a type of sustainable agriculture, the aim of organic farming can be expressed as a function of mini - max type: maximizing yields and minimizing the negative side effects of agricultural activities. Organic agriculture is a creation of farmers who love nature, as an alternative to intensive farming of industrial type, based on efficient production methods and means, in particular, economically.

In accordance with the Council Regulation (EC) 834/2007 and Commission Regulation (EC) 889/2008, EU countries use, with the same meaning, the terms of *organic agriculture* (England), *biological agriculture* (Greece, France, Italy, Netherlands and Portugal) and *ecological agriculture* (Denmark, Germany and Spain). Since 2000, Romania has been using the term organic farming, according to the regulations stipulated in the Emergency Ordinance 34/2000.

Organic farming emerged in Europe as a result of health problems and negative experiences caused by the use of synthetic chemicals generated by the intensive industrial technologies, based on the forcing of production by over-fertilization of agricultural land and the use of stimulators in animal nutrition. Organic farming is a dynamic sector that has experienced an upward trend, both in the plant and animal production sector. Respect for every living organism is a general principle of organic farming, from the smallest micro-organism from the ground up to the largest tree that grows above. Because of this, each step of the ecological chain is designed to maintain, and where possible, to increase the diversity of plants and animals. Improvement of biodiversity is often the result of good practices of organic agriculture, as well as respect for the EU Regulation on organic agricultural production [39; 40].

1.1. In the world

Worldwide, nearly 31 million hectares are used for organic production, representing 0.7% of the total agricultural land. This farming system is practiced in over 633 890 farms [38].

The regions with the largest areas of organically managed agricultural land are Oceania (12.1 million hectares of 33 % of the global organic farmland), Europe (10 million hectares of 27 % of the global organic farmland) and Latin America (8.4 million hectares or 23 %). The countries with the most organic agricultural land are Australia (12 million hectares), Argentina (4.2 million hectares) and the United States (1.9 million hectares). The highest shares of organic agricultural land are in the Falkland Islands (35.9 %), Liechtenstein (27.3 %) and Austria (19.7 %).

1.2. In Europe

According to the study of World of Organic Agriculture, seven of the first ten countries of the world, ranked by the percentage of the agricultural land cultivated in organic system, are in the European Union [38].

The area under organic agriculture has increased significantly in the last years. In the period 2000-2008, the total organic area has increased from 4.3 to an estimated 7.6 mio ha (+7.4% per year). The Member States with the largest areas in 2008 are Spain (1.13 mio ha), Italy (1.00 mio ha), Germany (0.91 mio ha), the United Kingdom (0.72 mio ha) and France (0.58 mio ha). As of the end of 2010, 10 million hectares in Europe were managed organically by almost 280'000 farms.

The countries in central and eastern Europe, like Poland, with areas of over 367,000 hectares cultivated organically and the Czech Republic, which had a market growth of 11% in 2009, are becoming increasingly important on the market of organic products [38].

Among arable crops, cereals represent the most important category with 1.2 mio ha in 2007, i.e. 18.3% of all EU organic land. The largest producers are Italy and Germany. Permanent grassland represents 2.51 mio ha (45.1% of the whole organic area and arable crops), in 2006. The higher level of permanent pastures in the organic sector stems from the more extensive production systems employed. In the EU-15, permanent pastures have represented more than 40% of all organic land. The area under permanent pastures is the highest in absolute terms in Germany, Spain and the United Kingdom where it is around 0.4 mio ha. In six Member States the organic sector amounts to more than 10% of the total area of permanent pastures: 25.8% in the Czech Republic, 16.0% in Greece, 16.2% in Latvia, 15.5% in Slovakia, 12.0% in Austria and 11.5% in Portugal.

Consumer food demand grows at a fast pace in the largest EU markets, yet the organic sector does not represent more than 2% of total food expenses in the EU- 15 in 2007 [38].

1.3. In Romania

In 2008, of the total area where organic farming was used, permanent pastures and forage crops represented 60,000 ha, the cereals 56,000 ha, oleaginous plants and protein plants 30,000 ha, while the collection and certification of plants and flowers from the spontaneous flora 59,000 ha. The data from 2011 show that the area cultivated organically was of about 300,000 ha. Of this area, the arable land occupies 158,825 ha, permanent grasslands and meadows 89,489 ha, permanent crops 54,840 ha, and the collection from spontaneous flora 47,101 ha [37].

Permanent grasslands, which are traditionally used as forage for ruminants, are an important land use in Europe and cover more than a third of the European agricultural area. In Europe extensive grazing by livestock and fertilization with their manure is considered an appropriate management strategy to conserve biodiversity value. The importance of permanent grasslands in Romania is shown by the area they occupy and by their comparatively high biodiversity. Currently, permanent pasture in Romania covers 4.9 million ha [37]. This area accounts for 33% of the total agricultural area of the country. In terms of area occupied by natural grasslands in Europe, Romania occupies fifth position after France, Britain, Spain and Germany. The permanent grasslands from Romania, situated on soils with low natural fertility, are weakly productive and have an improper flower composition. The main means for improving these grasslands consist in adjusting soil fertility, changing the dominance in the vegetal canopy and their good management. The organic fertilization and the rational use lead to substantial increases of the production, biodiversity and the fodder quality improvement. Increasing the productive potential of these grasslands can be achieved through fertilization with different rates and types of organic fertilizers. Previous studies have demonstrated the positive effects of organic fertilizers on grassland. Comparative studies, which investigated the effects of different management practices on grasslands, have demonstrated that changes do occur in species diversity and the composition of plant functional groups depending on management practices.

Each permanent grassland sward can be considered as a unique mixture of species at different growth stages and this complexity makes it difficult to characterize and understand their feed value. Floristic composition influences the nutritional value of permanent grasslands due to differences in the chemical composition, digestibility of individual species and variation in the growth rate of different species.

The problem of the biodiversity reached in the top of the actual preoccupations because the modern agriculture was lately focused on developing some methods and procedures to allow the management of a relatively restrained number of species, the immediate economic interest being primary, without making a deep analysis of the long and medium -term consequences. Often, the preoccupations concerning the productivity left no place for the quality of the products or for the environment's health.

The experience of the developed countries underlines the fact that taking decisions in the problem of biodiversity must be made only after conducting thorough, professional, interdisciplinary studies, which allow the projection of a sustainable management of the natural resources, among which the permanent pasture lands occupy an important place. Comparing the data from the specialty literature, regarding the Romania's pasture lands' vegetation from almost 40 years ago, we will observe that many of those aspects have modified. There are numerous technical solutions for making a compromise between the function of production of the meadows and maintaining their biodiversity.

2. Management of organic fertilizers

2.1. Importance of organic fertilizers

In the twentieth century numerous studies were made on the role of organic matter in defining soil fertility. Experimental fields were established in Rothamstead England (1843), Morrow, the U.S. (1876) Askov, Denmark (1894), Halle / Saale, Germany, Groningen, Netherlands, Dehéreim, France, Fundulea, Podu Iloaiei Suceava, Romania. The long-term experiments made in these fields contributed importantly to the knowledge of the effect of organic and mineral substances on improving soil fertility [20].

These long-term researches conducted worldwide established the utility of organic fertilizers for maintaining or increasing the organic component of the soil. The introduction of organic residues in soil means turning to good account the energy included in these livestock excreta. About 49% of the chemical energy contained in the organic compounds of the food consumed by animals is excreted as manure, where significant percentages of macro and micro- elements are to be found [20].

Consumption of organic products is a growing process, so agriculture must keep up and produce ever more. Obtaining products by producingno harmful effects to nature is almost impossible. One thing is sure, that farmers try to minimize these negative effects as much as possible.

Soil, which is the focus of organic farming, is considered a complex living environment, closely interacting with plants and animals. By its specific techniques, organic farming aims to increase the microbiological activity of the soil, to maintain and increase its fertility.

The organic substance used as fertilizer is an important component in order to maintain or restore the soil fertility. Collection, storage and fermentation of vegetal wastes so as to decrease their volume and improve their physicochemical properties are a requirement of organic farming.

For many considerations, the organic fertilizers are preferred in organic farming as poorly soluble nutrients are mobilized with the help of soil microorganisms.

Fertilization is an important means of increasing the amount of organic products and the methods of fertilization used vary from one farm to another. For fertilization, the natural fertilizers represented by animal or vegetal remains are used in organic farms.

The fertility and biological activity of the soil must be maintained and improved by the cultivation of legumes, green manure crops or deep-rooting plants in an appropriate rotation. Also, the fertility must be maintained by incorporating organic substances in the soil as compost or from the production units, which respect specific production rules.

Besides the use of legumes in rotations, the role of animals in the organic system facilitates nutrient recycling. The potential for recycling the nutrients through fertilizer application is high. Thus, both the nutrients from the grazing period and the nutrients from the stall period are concentrated in solid manure and urine which are available for redistribution. By grazing, the animals retain only 5-10% of the nitrogen existing in the grass consumed. Together with the manure, they remove about 70% of nitrogen in the urine and 30% in the solid manure.

Not all initial nitrogen in manure is used by herbs in the production of dry matter in the crop. Much of the nitrogen may be retained in roots, immobilized in organic matter in the soil or lost by leaching or denitrification. Also, the loss of nutrients during storage may occur due to leaching and volatilization, which depend largely on how these fertilizers are managed. The nitrogen losses as ammonia or nitrogen gas in the fertilizer can be of 10% of the total weight when it is tamped in the pile and reach 40% when the pile is loose and turned. The gaseous losses of urine can be of 10-20% and even higher when it is shaken. Because of this, the application in spring is more efficient because the leaching losses are lower than in the case of application in autumn or winter.

The organic fertilizers positively contribute to the modification of physical conditions in the soil by increasing the field capacity for water, aeration, porosity and brittleness, and the black colour of organic matter will lead to easier and faster heating of these soils [20].

It should be mentioned that, when using organic fertilizers it is very easy to overcome the nutrient dose that needs to be applied. Therefore, the amount applied for a complete rotation of the cultures should be limited to the equivalent of nutrient from the manure produced by maximum 2.5 to 3 units of cattle / ha.

2.2. Organic fertilizers used in Romania

2.2.1. Manure

The manure is composed of animal manure and bedding material, in variable amounts and in different stages of decomposition.

Because different types of bedding are used, in various amounts, and the animals are fed on different diets for long periods, the chemical composition of manure can vary widely.

In the aerobic composting of manure, the long time of composting increases the biological stability of the nitrogen compounds and the nitrogen availability decreases accordingly. Although the application of high doses of manure results in increasing the production of nitrogen, however the crops use less nitrogen of the manure applied in high doses.

The highest losses during waste storage are those occurring in gaseous form. The ammonia is lost each time the manure pile is moved, while inside the well compacted piles de-nitrifications can be caused due to the anaerobic conditions created. The losses by leaching from piles of uncovered manure can be considerable. The nitrogen losses by washing are reduced, being of only 4-6%, in case of the covered heaps, when compared to the losses of 10-14% in the case of unprotected piles [20].

The experiences showed that 60 to 90% of ammonia nitrogen from cattle manure can volatilize between the 5th and 25th day after the application on the soil surface. The losses by administration can be reduced by incorporating the manure in the soil as soon as possible. It should be noted that the standards of organic farming prohibit the use of manure derived from breeding systems, ethically unacceptable, such as batteries of cages and intensive poultry units.

There are two essential ways of approaching the manure management used in organic farming practices. The first approach involves the application of fresh manure in dose of about 10 t ha^{-1}. The alternative is the storage of manure in a wide range of possible conditions and its use in the moment it attained the over-maturation stage, but usually not later than six months.

Some farmers laid great emphasis on composting manure as a way of approaching the use of fresh manure, due to the microbiological activity associated with the decomposition occurring in the soil. The increased microbiological activity means that a larger amount of nutrients can be synthesized from the organic matter present in the soil.

During storage, several important chemical processes take place in the pile of manure. At first, the urea is converted into ammonia compounds, while carbohydrates from the bedding after the fermentation are converted into energy, different gases (e.g. CO_2, methane and hydrogen). At the same time, the proteins from the bedding are decomposed in simple nitrogen compounds and the nitrogen is assimilated and fixed by different bacteria.

A traditional approach to storing manure in central Europe is the "cold manure" technique, where the manure is carefully stored and compacted, thus creating complete conditions of anaerobiosis. However large losses are recorded during administration, because the material must be left at the soil surface for the toxic products synthesized during fermentation not to prevent root growth and microbiological processes from the soil.

The careful control of the conditions in which the decomposition takes place allows the decomposition process to be optimized. The microbiological activity increases rapidly at temperatures around 60°C, and after a few weeks the pile is turned over to allow a second heating.

The high temperatures developed during composting help destroy the weed seeds and pathogens. The insects present in compost will eat the eggs of cabbage root fly, but the problem can be solved only if the distribution of compost is made in the adequate stage of fly development [20].

This is one of the reasons why the standards of organic agriculture recommend manure be composted before use.

In Britain, large quantities of organic fertilizers are produced on stubble, where their accumulation is allowed for a certain period of time. In case the composting was made too strongly it results a paste that can be used only when it corresponds to the proposed specific goals.

2.2.2. *Vinassa*

Vinassa is a by-product obtained after the evaporation of waste waters from factories that produce bakery yeast [11]. The waste waters from production, after the separation of yeast from the culture medium, represented by molasses derived from sugar factories, are subjected to concentration by evaporation, turning into a valuable product called vinasse, CMS (Condensed molasses solubles) FEL (Fermentation end Liquor), Dickschlempe). The vinassa product looks like a dark brown liquid, with relatively low viscosity, caramel odor slightly unpleasant because of the presence of phenols and sweet bitter taste.

Vinassa has a very low level of fermentable sugars (1.5 to 2.0%), and the product is very stable in time and does not have storage problems. The valuable composition of vinasse makes it widely used in western Europe as an organic fertilizer, encapsulating material for fertilizers and feed additive for ruminants, pigs and poultry [6; 21; 32].

Quality ratios	U.M.	Average values	Quality indexes	U.M.	Average values
Dry matter	%	61-63	Zinc	mg/100g	0,5-0,6
Humidity	%	39-37	Organic carbon	%	18,26
Sugars	%	1,5-2	Lactic acid	%	1,28-1,29
Raw protein	%	18-21	Formic acid	%	0,001-0,011
Ash	%	21-23	Acetic acid	%	0,47-0,475
Potassium	%	5-7	Malic acid	%	0,28-0,281
Calcium	%	0,99-1,1	Glucose	%	0,04-0,044
Magnesium	%	0,11-0,12	Fructose	%	0,05-0,06
Sodium	%	6-6,2	Betaine	%	13,3-14,5
Phosphor	%	0,3-0,5	Glycerin	%	2,03-2,07
Nitrites	%	0,005-0,006	Total nitrogen	%	2,8-3,2
Nitrates	%	0,8-1,1	Free amino acids		
Ph		7-8	glutamic acid	g/kg	4,57-4,76
Iron	mg/100g	27-30	methionine	g/kg	0,08-1,29
Copper	mg/100g	0,60-0,65	lysine	g/kg	1,1-1,6

Table 1. Chemical composition of vinassa [32].

Vinassa has a complex chemical composition (Table 1), being rich in total nitrogen (3.0 to 3.2%), very rich in potassium (5-7%) and low in phosphorus (0.3 to 0.5 %). It also contains appreciable quantities of sodium (6.0 to 6.2%), calcium (0.99 to 1.1%), magnesium (0.11 to 0.12%), iron (27-30 mg / 100 g soil), copper (0.60 to 0.65 mg/100 g soil) and zinc (from 0.50 to 0.60 mg/100 g soil) etc.

Due to its chemical composition, vinassa leads to the formation of bacterial flora in the soil which accelerates the degradation of cellulose material and enables fast incorporation in the natural circuit of vegetal residues in the cellulose material. This property recommends vinassa for use in direct spraying on the stubbles left after harvesting the cereals. In addition, because of the high content in potassium and nitrogen, vinassa is considered a valuable organic fertilizer.

Following the research carried out, the product was approved in 2003 as the vinassa-Rompak or just "vinassa". Used in dilution with water in 1:5 ratio on permanent pastures, "vinassa" reacts as a semi-organic fertilizer, with beneficial effects on productivity and quality of the forage. An important role of "vinassa" is also present in the formation of bacterial flora responsible for the degradation of cellulose material in the soil and due to its content of potassium and nitrogen it can replace totally or partially the application of mineral fertilizers.

3. Organic fertilizers used on permanent grasslands: an example of Romania

3.1. Manure used on *Festuca valesiaca* and *Agrostis capillaris+Festuca rubra* grasslands

The experiment has investigated the influence of organic fertilizers, applied each year or every 2-3 years, at rates of 10-30 t ha^{-1}, in a *Festuca valesiaca* grassland, situated at the height of 107 m, at Ezareni-Iasi County, and at rates of 10-30 t ha^{-1}, in an *Agrostis capillaris+Festuca rubra* grassland, situated at the height of 707 m at Pojorata-Suceava County, on yield and flower composition. Even if permanent grasslands from north-eastern Romania are found at a rate of 70% on fields affected by erosion, which highly diminishes their productive potential, the most important reduction in their productivity is due to unfavourable climatic conditions and bad management [29; 30]. Increasing the grassland productive potential can be achieved by different fertilization rates and types of organic fertilizers [2; 28]. The investigations carried out until today have demonstrated the positive effects of manure on grasslands and, if applied reasonably, it can replace all the chemical fertilizers [15; 33].

These trials was set up at two different sites: Ezareni – Iasi site, from the forest steppe area, on a *Festuca valesiaca* L. grassland, and Pojorata – Suceava site, on *Agrostis capillaris + Festuca rubra* grassland, from the boreal floor; both sites present a weak botanical composition. The trial from Ezareni – Iasi was set up at the height of 107 m, on 18-20% slope, and the one from Pojorata – Suceava, at the height of 707 m, on 20% slope. The climatic conditions were characterized by mean temperatures of 9.5 0C and total rainfall amounts of 552.4 mm at Ezareni – Iasi, and by mean temperatures of 6.3 ^{0}C and total rainfall amounts of 675 mm at Pojorata - Suceava. An important fact was that the year 2007 was very dry at Ezareni – Iasi, and the climatic conditions were unfavourable to the good development of vegetation on grasslands.

Analyzing the production data concerning the *Festuca valesiaca* grassland from Ezareni, we have noticed that in 2006, they were comprised between 1.56 t ha^{-1} DM at the control and 2.71 t ha^{-1} DM at the fertilization with 40 t ha^{-1} cattle manure, applied every 3 years (Table 2). The highest yields were found in case of 40 t ha^{-1} manure fertilization, applied every 3 years; the yields were of 2.57 t ha^{-1} DM in case of sheep manure and 2.71 t ha^{-1} DM in case of cattle manure. In 2007, the vegetation from permanent grasslands was highly affected by the long-term draught that dominated the experimental area from Ezareni, since September 2006 until August 2007, so that the productivity of these agro-ecosystems was greatly diminished, the effect of fertilization on production becoming negligible. The mean yields during 2006-2007 were comprised between 1.09 t ha^{-1} DM at the control and 1.96 t ha^{-1} DM in case of fertilization with 40 t ha^{-1} cattle manure, every 3 years.

Fertilization variant	2006	2007	Average
V_1 . Unfertilized control	1.56	0.61	1.09
V_2 . 10 t ha^{-1} sheep manure applied every year	2.16	0.91	1.54*
V_3 . 20 t ha-1 sheep manure applied every 2 years	2.35	1.02	1.69**
V_4 . 30 t ha^{-1} sheep manure applied every 3 years	2.12	1.01	1.57**
V_5 . 40 t ha^{-1} sheep manure applied every 3 years	2.57	1.12	1.85***
V_6 . 10 t ha^{-1} cattle manure	2.28	1.13	1.71**
V_7 . 20 t ha^{-1} cattle manure applied every 2 years	2.50	1.09	1.80***
V_8 . 30 t ha^{-1} cattle manure applied every 3 years	2.69	1.04	1.87***
V_9 . 40 t ha^{-1} cattle manure applied every 3 years	2.71	1.21	1.96***
Average	2.33	1.02	1.68

**=P≤0.05; **=P≤0.01; ***=P≤0.001; NS= not significant*

Table 2. Influence of organic fertilization on DM yield (t ha^{-1}), Ezareni, Iasi [29].

In the trial conducted on the *Agrostis capillaris+Festuca rubra* grassland from Pojorata in 2006, the yields were between 2.95 t ha^{-1} DM at the control and 4.17 t ha^{-1} DM at 30 Mg ha^{-1} manure fertilization, applied every 3 years (Table 3). In 2007, the yields were higher than in 2006, being comprised between 4.34 t ha^{-1} at the control and 5.51 t ha^{-1} in case of fertilization with 30 t ha^{-1} manure, applied every 3 years. The mean yields during 2006-2007 have been influenced by climate and the type and level of organic fertilization, being comprised between 3.65 t ha^{-1} at the control and 4.84 t ha^{-1} in case of fertilization with 30 t ha^{-1} manure, applied every 3 years.

The analysis of canopy has shown that the mean values of the presence rate were of 68% in grasses, 13% in legumes and 19% in other species (Table 4) and 39% in grasses, 32% in legumes and 29% in other species (Table 5).

Fertilization variant	2006	2007	Average
Unfertilized control	2.95	4.34	3.65
10 t ha^{-1} cattle manure applied every year	3.50	5.05	4.28**
20 t ha-1 cattle manure applied every 2 years	3.90	4.90	4.40**
30 t ha^{-1} cattle manure applied every 3 years	4.17	5.51	4.84***
20 t ha^{-1} cattle manure applied in the first year+10 t ha^{-1} cattle manure applied in the second year+0 t ha^{-1} manure applied in the third year	3.86	4.87	4.37**
20 t ha^{-1} cattle manure applied in the first year+0 t ha^{-1} manure applied in the second year+10 t ha^{-1} cattle manure applied in the third year	3.78	5.25	4.52**
20 t ha^{-1} cattle manure applied in the first year+10 t ha^{-1} cattle manure applied in the second year+10 t ha^{-1} cattle manure applied in the third year	4.03	4.81	4.42**
10 t ha^{-1} cattle manure applied in the first year+20 t ha^{-1} cattle manure applied in the second year+10 t ha^{-1} cattle manure applied in the third year	3.63	5.12	4.38**
Average	3.72	4.98	4.36**

**=P≤0.05; **=P≤0.01; ***=P≤0.001; NS= not significant*

Table 3. Influence of organic fertilization on DM yield (t ha^{-1}), Pojorata, Suceava [30].

At Ezareni – Iasi, a total number of 40 species was registered, of which 6 species from grass family, 10 species from Fabaceae and 24 species from others, while at Pojorata – Suceava, the total number of species was of 45, of which 12 grasses, 9 legumes and 24 species from others. The species with the highest presence rate from Ezareni – Iasi were *Festuca valesiaca* (39%), *Trifolium pratense* (7%), *Plantago media* (3%), *Achillea setacea* (4%), and from Pojorata – Suceava, *Agrostis capillaris* (14%), *Festuca rubra* (7%), *Trisetum flavescens* (6%), *Trifolium repens* (16%), *Trifolium pratense* (8%) and *Taraxacum officinale* (5%).

Fertilization variant	Grass	Legumes	Other species
Unfertilized control	69	10	21
10 t ha^{-1} sheep manure applied every year	76	13	11
20 t ha-1 sheep manure applied every 2 years	59	16	25
30 t ha^{-1} sheep manure applied every 3 years	70	11	19
40 t ha^{-1} sheep manure applied every 3 years	67	15	18
10 t ha^{-1} cattle manure	62	11	27
20 t ha^{-1} cattle manure applied every 2 years	68	16	16
30 t ha^{-1} cattle manure applied every 3 years	71	12	17
40 t ha^{-1} cattle manure applied every 3 years	69	11	20
Average	68	13	19

Table 4. Influence of the organic fertilization on the canopy structure (%), Ezareni, Iasi [30].

Fertilization variant	Grass	Legumes	Other species
Unfertilized control	44	25	31
10 t ha^{-1} manure applied every year	38	33	29
20 t ha-1 manure applied every 2 years	43	30	27
30 t ha^{-1} manure applied every 3 years	37	33	30
20 t ha^{-1} manure applied in the first year+10 t ha^{-1} manure applied in the second year+0 t ha^{-1} manure applied in the third year	36	36	28
20 t ha^{-1} manure applied in the first year+0 t ha^{-1} manure applied in the second year+10 t ha^{-1} manure applied in the third year	42	30	28
20 t ha^{-1} manure applied in the first year+10 t ha^{-1} manure applied in the second year+10 t ha^{-1} manure applied in the third year	36	33	31
10 t ha^{-1} manure applied in the first year+20 t ha^{-1} manure applied in the second year+10 t ha^{-1} manure applied in the third year	33	37	30
Average	39	32	29

Table 5. Influence of the organic fertilization on the canopy structure (%), Pojorata, Suceava [30].

The yields obtained were influenced in both experiencing sites by climatic conditions, type and level of organic fertilization. Our results demonstrated the positive effects of organic fertilizers on canopy structure, biodiversity and productivity in the studied permanent grasslands. In both trials, we noticed that the highest number of species (24 species) was represented by others, proving that the management of organic fertilizers did not affect the biodiversity of these grassland types.

3.2. Manure used on *Nardus stricta* L. Grasslands in Romania's Carpathians

In Romania, the grassland area, dominated by *Nardus stricta* L., covers 200,000 hectares. Meadow degradation is determined by changes that take place in plant living conditions and in the structure of vegetation. For a long-term period no elementary management measures were applied on permanent meadows in Romania, estimating that they could get efficient yields without technological inputs. The organic fertilization has a special significance for permanent meadows if their soils show some unfavourable chemical characteristics. The investigations carried out until today have demonstrated the positive effects of reasonably applied manure on grasslands. Within this context, the main aim of our study was to improve the productivity of natural grasslands by finding economically efficient solutions that respect their sustainable use and the conservation of biodiversity [1; 17; 31]. On the other hand, the productivity and fodder quality are influenced by the floristic composition, morphological characteristics of plants, grassland management, vegetation stage at harvest and level of fertilization [1; 4; 8; 34].

To accomplish the objectives of these studies we have conducted an experiment in the Cosna region, in four repetitions blocks with 20 sq. meter randomized plots on *Nardus stricta* L.

grasslands, situated at an altitude of 840 m, on districambosol with 1.36 mg/100 g soil PAL and 38.1 mg/100 g soil KAL [13].

The forage obtained from these grasslands is mainly used to feed dairy cows. The influence of manure has been analysed, and applied each year or every two years at rates of 20-50 t ha^{-1} (table 6). The manure with a content of 0.42% total N, 0.19% $_{P2O5}$ and 0.27% K_2O was applied by hand, early in spring, at the beginning of grass growth. The Kjeldahl method was used for the determination of crude protein, the Weende method for the determination of crude fiber, the photometrical method for the determination of total phosphorus, ash was determined by ignition, whereas the nitrogen nutrition index (NNI) was determined by the method developed by Lemaire et al. (1989): $NNI=100 \times N/4,8 \times (DM)^{-0,32}$, where N: plant nitrogen content (%), DM: dry mater production (t ha^{-1}). All fodder analyses have been performed on samples taken from the first harvest cycle, based on the average values of the years 2009-2010. The vegetation was studied using the method Braun-Blanquét. For floristic data were calculated the mean abundance-dominance (ADm). Data regarding the sharwe of economic groups, species number and Shannon Index (SI) were processed by analysis of variance.

The use of 20-50 t ha^{-1} manure accounted for, alongside the climatic factors, a significant yield increase, especially when applying 30-50 t ha^{-1}. At these rates, the DM yield recorded a significant increase, compared with the control variant. Considering the average of the two years, the control variant recorded values of 1.77 t ha^{-1}, whereas by fertilization, we obtained yields of 3.29-5.53 t ha-1 DM, at rates of 30-50 t ha^{-1}, applied on a yearly basis, and 2.86-3.33 t ha^{-1} DM at the same rates, applied once every 2 years, respectively (Table 6).

Manure rate	**2009**	**2010**	**Average of 2009-2010**	
	t ha^{-1}	t ha^{-1}	t ha^{-1}	%
Unfertilized control	1.25	2.30	1.77	100
20 t ha^{-1}, every year	2.55*	2.40	2.48ns	140
30 t ha^{-1}, every year	2.34*	4.23**	3.29**	186
40 t ha^{-1}, every year	3.59***	4.74***	4.17***	236
50 t ha^{-1}, every year	4.73***	6.32***	5.53***	312
20 t ha^{-1}, every 2 years	2.28 ns	2.92 ns	2.60 ns	147
30 t ha^{-1}, every 2 years	2.59*	3.13 ns	2.86*	162
40 t ha^{-1}, every 2 years	1.78	4.14**	2.96*	167
50 t ha^{-1}, every 2 years	2.39*	4.28**	3.33**	188

**=P≤0.05; **=P≤0.01; ***=P≤0.001; ns= not significant*

Table 6. Influence of organic fertilization on the yield (t ha^{-1} DM) of *Nardus stricta* grasslands from the Carpathian Mountains of Romania [34].

The organic fertilization of *Nardus stricta* L. grasslands, with moderate rates of 20–30 t ha^{-1} manure, has determined the increase in the CP (crude protein) content by 45.9 g kg^{-1} DM, compared with the unfertilized control variant. The rates of 40-50 t ha^{-1} diminished the percentage of dominant species and the increase of CP yield with 246.2-422.8 kg ha^{-1} when manure was added once a year and 189.0-243.2 kg ha^{-1}, when manure was added every 2 years, respectively, in comparison with the control variant (Table 7). The ash content increased in all fertilized soils, varying between 71.0–83.1 g kg^{-1} DM, compared to merely 61.2 g kg^{-1} DM at the control variant. The crude fiber content (CF) was the highest at the control variant (285.3 g kg^{-1} DM) and the lowest at the variant fertilized with 50 t ha-1, applied once every 2 years, of 228.3 g kg^{-1} DM. Phosphorus, an important element in animal nutrition, recorded an increase from 1.4 g kg^{-1} DM at the control to 2.2 g kg^{-1} DM with the use 50 t ha^{-1} manure, applied once every 2 years (table 2). The NNI presented values comprised between 25-53, thus, indicating a deficiency in nitrogen nutrition.

Manure rate	t ha^{-1} DM	CP	Ash	CF	P_{total}	Kg ha^{-1} CP	NNI
Unfertilized control	1.77	62.6	61.2	285.3	1.41	110.8	25
20 t ha^{-1}, every year	2.48	88.2***	71.0	264.2	1.92*	218.7	39
30 t ha^{-1}, every year	3.29**	108.5***	83.1	270.4	2.05*	357.0	53
40 t ha^{-1}, every year	4.17***	97.9***	78.2	258.1	2.13**	408.2	52
50 tg ha^{-1}, every year	5.53***	96.5***	81.6	253.6	2.04*	533.6	55
20 t ha^{-1}, every 2 years	2.60	82.8***	79.0	247.5	1.86*	215.3	37
30 t ha^{-1}, every 2 years	2.86*	92.2***	77.5	241.6	2.17*	263.7	43
40 t ha^{-1}, every 2 years	2.96*	101.3***	80.7	230.5	1.95*	299.8	48
50 t ha^{-1}, every 2 years	3.33**	106.3***	79.2	228.3	2.22**	354.0	52

* $P \leq 0.05$; ** $P \leq 0.01$; *** $P \leq 0.001$
CP=crude protein, CF=crude fiber, P_{total}= total phosphorus, NNI= nitrogen nutrition index

Table 7. Influence of organic fertilization on yield (t ha^{-1} DM) and NNI and CP quantity (Kg ha^{-1}) and on chemical composition of the fodder obtained from *Nardus stricta* grasslands (g kg^{-1} DM), mean 2009-2010 [34].

The organic fertilization on permanent grasslands has resulted in some changes in the canopy structure, both in terms of the number of species as well as in their percentage in the vegetal canopy [4; 8; 16; 22; 24; 34]. Thus, the number of species has increased from 18 at the control variant to 25-31 at fertilization rates, while the percentage of *Nardus stricta* L. species plunged from 70% at the control to 14-33% in the case of the fertilized experiments. Moreover, the legume species increased by 5-28% (Table 8a).

Species number increased towards the control,for all fertilization variants. Shannon weaver index (SI) was compared to the control with the value between 1.07 and 2.52 (Table 8b).

Biodiversity has become one of the main concerns of our world, because modern farming, forestry and meadow culture focussed, in these latter years, on developing methods and proceedings for achieving high productions, without being interested in the quality of produces or environment health. Among the factors threatening biodiversity, one enlists human activities, high pressures on natural resources, division, change or even destruction of habitats, excessive use of pesticides, chemical fertilizers etc [36]. Nowadays, many specialists are concerned with adapting the technologies of fodder production to the new economic and ecological requirements, whilst the maintaining of biodiversity occupies an important place [3; 5; 9; 10; 14; 25; 35].

Species	**Plant ADm[1] degree %**								
	V_1	**V_2**	**V_3**	**V_4**	**V_5**	**V_6**	**V_7**	**V_8**	**V_9^2**
Agrostis capillaries	+	5	3	2	1	+	+	+	5
Anthoxanthum odoratum	-	4	+	-	+	3	6	4	5
Briza media	+	6	6	5	6	8	7	8	10
Cynosurus cristatus	-	-	-	-	-	3	+	-	-
Dactilys glomerata	-	-	-	-	3	-	-	-	-
Festuca pratensis	-	+	10	6	2	-	-	2	-
Festuca rubra	+	1	+	3	3	+	5	5	3
Nardus stricta	70	32	15	14	15	41	32	33	31
Phleum pretense	+	7	2	-	-	-	-	-	2
Grasses	***70***	***55***	***36***	***30***	***30***	***55***	***50***	***52***	***56***
Lotus corniculatus	-	18	13	2	3	5	5	5	+
Trifolium pretense	+	10	5	3	5	3	4	3	5
Trifolium repens	-	+	+	-	+	2	3	2	+
Legumes	***0***	***28***	***18***	***5***	***8***	***10***	***12***	***10***	***5***
Achillea millefolium	+	3	12	35	40	20	9	6	5
Ajuga reptans	+	+	+	+	+	+	+	+	+
Alchemilla xanthochlora	6	2	6	2	6	3	6	3	6
Chrysanthemum leucanthemum	2	3	-	-	-	-	-	-	-
Campanula obietina	-	+	+	+	+	+	+	2	4
Centaurea cyanus	-	-	+	-	-	-	-	-	-
Cerastium semidecandrum	1	+	+	+	+	+	5	3	+
Cruciata glabra	2	2	3	+	3	+	+	3	3
Fragaria vesca	-	-	+	+	+	+	+	+	+
Hyeracium pilosella	3	2	3	+	-	+	-	+	+
Hypericum maculatum	2	+	1	3	2	2	4	6	6
Leucanthemum vulgare	-	-	+	-	-	-	-	-	+
Luzula multiflora	-	-	-	-	-	+	+	-	-

http://dx.doi.org/10.5772/52006

Species	Plant ADm[1] degree %								
	V_1	V_2	V_3	V_4	V_5	V_6	V_7	V_8	V_9[2]
Lychnis flos-cuculi	-	-	+	+	+	+	-	-	-
Prunella vulgaris	+	+	+	+	-	+	+	-	+
Polygala amarelle	-	-	-	-	-	-	+	-	-
Polygala vulgaris	-	-	-	-	+	+	-	-	-
Plantago lanceolata	-	-	+	+	3	+	+	2	+
Potentila ternate	5	4	5	+	4	5	-	2	2
Rumex acetosa	-	-	-	-	-	+	-	+	-
Rumex acetosella	-	1	+	-	+	1	+	-	-
Ranunculus acer	1	-	+	2	2	1	+	2	+
Taraxacum officinale	2	0	2	+	+	3	4	4	-
Thymus pulegioides	2	-	2	-	-	+	+	+	-
Tragopogon pratensis	-	+	-	-	-	+	+	-	+
Veronica chamaedrys	1	+	12	+	-	-	10	5	1
Veronica officinalis	1	-	-	23	2	-	-	-	7
Viola tricolor	2	+	+	+	-	+	+	+	5
Forbs	***30***	***17***	***46***	***65***	***62***	***35***	***38***	***38***	***39***
Number of species	18	25	30	25	26	31	28	26	27
Shannon Index (SI)	1.07	2.27*	2.52*	1.93	2.15*	1.96	2.28*	2.50*	2.41*

[1] *ADm – mean abundance-dominance;*
[2] *V_1 is control, V_2-V_9 are the manure rates applied; *= P<0.05, ** = P<0.1, ***= P<0.01*

Table 8. Influence of organic fertilization on the evolution of the vegetal canopy, [34].

Previous research, done in different climatic and managerial conditions proved that there is a relationship between biodiversity and pastures productivity. The latter is influenced by the soils fertility, chemical reaction, and usage, intensity of grazing, altitude, amount and distribution rainfalls [7; 12; 18; 19; 23; 31].

The management applied on oligotrophic grasslands from Garda de Sus (Apuseni Mountain) is a traditional one. The maintenance activities ar only manually performed, among them the fertilization with stable manure being the most important one [26]. The grassland type of the untreated witness is *Agrostis capillaris* L *Festuca rubra* L The productivity of the respective meadows is very low, situation wich explains one of the reasons for the abandonment of oligotrophic grasslands in the area.

The low yield can be explained through the reduced quantities of rainfall from spring and through the reduced trophicity of the soil. The species diversity ot the studied phytocenosis is medium, and the number of species ranges from 20 up 24.

The floristic structure of the trated variants is significantly correlated with the general cover. The administration of technological inouts produces a considerable decrease of the phyto-diversity, especially in case of the variants treated with larger quantities of fertilizers [27].

3.3. Vinassa used as a fertilizer on *Festuca valesiaca* grassland

The objective of this study was to identify new opportunities to improve the permanent grassland, using "vinassa" as a fertilizer. The experiment was conducted on a permanent pasture of *Festuca valesiaca*, located on a land with a slope of 7-11% in 2000. The soil was of cambic chernozem type with loam-clay texture, low leachated with pH values from 6.5 to 7.1. The content in mobile phosphorus (P_{AL}) was of 28-46 ppm, mobile potassium (K_{AL}) of 333-400 ppm, the humus of 3.22-4.85% and total nitrogen (N_t) of 0.6-1.25, in the layer of 0-20 cm. The administration of the by-product was made after the dilution with water in 1:5 ratio and the way of using lawn was that of a grassland.

During the three years of study, there was a steady increase in dry matter production (Table 9). The meadow of *Festuca valesiaca* positively reacted to the use of "vinassa" by-product in normal vegetation conditions. The exception was 2002, when due to bad weather conditions, mainly water shortages in spring, the productions recorded a slight decrease in comparison with 2000.

Thus, in 2000, the production, in variants with total application of the sub-product in spring, ranged from 3.35 t ha^{-1} DM in the control sample and 3.99 t ha^{-1} DM, to 7 t ha^{-1} "vinassa". In 2000, in the variants with fractional application of fertilizers, the productions ranged from 3.07 t ha^{-1} in the control samples and 4.15 t ha^{-1} at 5 t ha^{-1}. 2001 was characterized by increased lawn productivity in both applications of vinassa, with increased production for the variants of full implementation in spring when the average productions were 5.97 t ha^{-1} in the control sample and 10.86 t ha^{-1} at 7 t ha^{-1} "vinassa".

In 2002 the recorded productions were lower than in 2001, due to less favorable weather conditions. In 2002 we noticed that the uneven distribution of rainfall during the vegetation period, that is heavy rains in the second half of the year, positively influenced the production increases, especially in the variants with fractional application.

The analysis of the average productions obtained in the three years shows that "vinassa" sub-product had a positive effect on the productivity of meadows, but also the results were conditioned by the climatic factors. In comparison to the control sample, in the case of vinassa with total application in spring, the production increased between 23 and 69% (2 t ha^{-1} "vinassa" and 7 t ha^{-1} "vinassa"), being statistically ensured, while the fractional application yielded smaller increases of 13-39% (2 t ha^{-1} "vinassa" and 7 t ha^{-1} "vinassa").

Using the "vinassa" sub-product as nitrogen-potassium fertilizer on permanent meadows of Festuca valesiaca L. determines production increase, statistically ensured of 23-69% (2 t ha^{-1} "vinassa" and 7 t ha^{-1} "vinassa") at total application in spring and 13-46% in fractionated administration (2 t ha^{-1} "vinassa").

http://dx.doi.org/10.5772/52006

Period	Variant	2000	2001	2002	Average 2000-2002	
		t ha^{-1}	t ha^{-1}	t ha^{-1}	t ha^{-1}	%
a_1	1	3.35	5.97	4.94	4.75	100
	2	3.36	8.06	6.65	6.02*	123
	3	3.44	8.39	7.04	6.29*	132
	4	3.69	8.54	7.11	6.45*	136
	5	3.59	9.24	8.47	7.10**	149
	6	3.76	10.07	9.48	7.77***	164
	7	3.99	10.86	9.17	8.01***	169
Average		3.93	8.92	7.95	6.93	146
a_2	1	3.07	5.97	5.17	4.74	100
	2	3.24	5.49	7.40	5.38 ns	113
	3	3.47	5.59	7.94	5.67 ns	120
	4	3.60	5.63	8.06	5.76 ns	122
	5	4.15	5.86	8.47	6.16 ns	130
	6	3.80	6.08	9.48	6.45*	136
	7	3.90	6.16	9.67	6.58*	139
Average		3.63	6.18	8.28	6.03	127

**=P≤0.05; **=P≤0.01; ***=P≤0.001; ns= not significant*

Table 9. Influence of vinassa on production of dry matter a meadow of *Festuca valesiaca* [32].

4. Conclusions

Organic farming is a dynamic sector in Romania recording an upward trend, both in the vegetal and animal production sector in recent years.

One of the essential conditions for the development of organic farming is to promote the concept of organic farming so as to make the consumer aware of the benefits of organic food consumption.

The fertilization of mountain grasslands with organic fertilizers leads to an improvement in terms biodiversity, productivity and quality.

Fertilization with manure contributed to the improvement of the botanical structure by increasing the percent of grasses, thus disfavouring the leguminous plants. The used management, characterized in time by low inputs and stability, has contributed to obtaining rather high productions and conservation of the biodiversity of the meadows from Romania.

The highest biodiversity was found in the grassland from Pojorata, covered with 45 species of Agrostis capillaris + Festuca rubra, compared to 40 species found in the grassland from Ezareni, covered with Festuca valesiaca.

The fertilization of *Nardus stricta* grasslands with 20-50 Mg ha-1 manure influenced the yield increase by 40-212% and brought along important changes in the chemical composition of fodder, improving its quality significantly, by increasing the CP content from 62.6 g kg^{-1} DM (control) to 108.5 (30 Mg ha^{-1} manure, applied once every 2 years); the total phosphorus from 1.41 to 2.22 g kg^{-1} DM and ash from 61.2 to 83.1 g kg^{-1}, and by diminishing the CF content from 285.3 to 228.3 g kg^{-1} DM, thus increasing fodder digestibility.

The application of 20-50 Mg ha^{-1} manure determined important changes in the flower composition as well, by lowering the percentage of *Nardus stricta* species from 70% to 14-33% and increasing the percentage of legumes (*Lotus corniculatus, Trifolium pratense* and *Trifolium repens*) and forbs.

The administration of "vinassa" sub-product in doses of 4-7 t ha^{-1} by 1:5 dilution with water does not determine spectacular increases in the production of DM.

In quantitative terms we noticed that, when fractioning, the vinassa production was lower than in variants with total application in spring, this being also caused by less favorable climatic conditions.

The period of vinassa application, the dosage used and the climatic conditions affect the productivity of permanent meadows. The best results were obtained when using doses of 6-7 t ha^{-1} "vinassa", with total application in spring (7.65 - 8.01 t ha^{-1} DM).

The results presented in this study, on land considered to be regionally representative of large parts of the Romania, indicated that fertilization treatments were able to maintain a high diversity of species. Production was influenced by climatic conditions, fertilizer application rate and the combination fertilizers applied. Using a low input-based management system can be a solution that will lead to higher yields and contribute to biodiversity conservation.

Author details

Samuil Costel * and Vintu Vasile

*Address all correspondence to: csamuil@uaiasi.ro

University of Agricultural Sciences and Veterinary Medicine in Iasi, Romania

References

[1] Bullock, J. M., Pywell, R. F., & Walker, K. J. (2007). Long-term enhancement of agricultural production by restoration of biodiversity. *Journal of applied ecology*, 44(1), 6-12.

[2] Cardaşol, V. (1994). Fertilisation organique des prairies permanentes roumaines; synthese des résultats d'essais multilocaux et de longue durée. *Revue Fourrages*, 139, 383-390.

[3] Duelli, P. (1997). Biodiversity evaluation in agricultural landscapes: An approach at two different scales. *Agriculture, Ecosystems and Environment*, 62(2-3), 81-91.

[4] Duru, M., Cruz, P., & Theau, J. P. (2010). A simplifies for characteristing agronomic services provided by species-rich grasslands. *Crop and pasture science*, 61(5), 420-433.

[5] Elsaesser, M., Kunz, H. G., & Briemle, G. (2008). Strategy of organic fertilizer use on permanent grassland- results of a 22-year-old experiment on meadow and mowing-pasture. *Grassland Science in Europe*, 13, 580-582.

[6] Haden, A., & Jourmet, M. (1980). Aliments liquides a base de vinasse de levurerie et sans urée pour compléter les rations de fourages pauvres distribuées a des genisses d'élevage". *Bull. Tech. C.R.Z.V.-Teix, INRA*, France.

[7] Hector, A., & Loreau, M. (2005). Relationships between biodiversity and production in grasslands at local and regional scales. *Grassland: A Global Resource, Editor McGilloway D.A.*, 295-304.

[8] Hejcman, M., Szakova, J., Schellberg, J., & Tlustos, P. (2010). The Rengen Grassland Experiment: relatioship between soil and biomass chemical properties, amount of elements applied, and their uptake. *Plant and soil*, 333(1-2), 163-179.

[9] Hejcman, M., Klaudisova, M., Schellberg, J., & Honsova, D. (2007). The Rengen Grassland Experiment: Plant species composition after 64 years of fertilizer application. *Agriculture ecosystems and environment*, 122, 259-266.

[10] Hopkins, A., Pywell, R. F., Peel, S., Johnson, R. H., & Bowling, P. J. (1999). Enhancement of botanical diversity of permanent grassland and impact on hay production in Environmentally Sensitive Areas in the UK. *Grass and Forage Science*, 54, 163-173.

[11] Ionel, A., Vintu, V., Halga, P., & Samuil, C. (2000). Vinasse"- fertilizant şi aditiv furajer. *Lucrări ştiinţifice*, 43-44, Seria Zootehnie, Editura "Ion Ionescu de la Brad" Iaşi, 862-866.

[12] Isselstein, J., Griffith, B. A., Pradel, P., & Venerus, S. (2007). Effects of livestock breed and grazing intensity on biodiversity and production in grazing systems. Nutritive value of herbage and livestock performance. *Grass and Forage Science*, 62(2), 145-158.

[13] Janssens, F., Peeters, A., Tallowin, J. R. B., Bakker, J. P., Bekker, R. M., Fillat, F., & Oomes, M. J. M. (1998). Relationship between soil chemical factors and grassland diversity. *Plant and soil*, 202(1), 69-78.

[14] Jeangros, B. (2002). Peut-on augmenter la diversité botanique d'une prairie permanente en supprimant la fumure? *Revue Suisse d'Agriculture*, 34(6), 287-292.

[15] Jeangros, B., Sahli, A., & Jacot, P. (2003). Une fumure organique a-t-elle le même effet qu ´une fumure minerale sur une prairie permanente. *Revue suisse d'Agriculture*, 35(4).

[16] Kirkham, F. W., Tallowin, J. R. B., Sanderson, R. A., Bhogal, A., Chambers, B. J., & Stevens, D. P. (2008). The impact of organic and inorganic fertilizers and lime on the species-richness and lant functional characteristics of hay meadow communities. *Biological conservation*, 141(5), 1411-1427.

[17] Klavina, D., Adamovics, A., & Straupe, I. (2001). Botanical composition and productivity of meadows in Tervete Nature Park. *Conference on sustainable agriculture in Baltic States*, proceedings, 54-56.

[18] Kopec, M., Zarzycki, J., & Gondek, K. (2010). Species diversity of submontane grasslands: effects of topographic and soil factors. *Polish Journal of Ecology*, 58(2), 285-295.

[19] Lampkin, N. (1999). *Organic farming*, Farming press.

[20] Lixandru, G., & Filipov, F. (2012). *Ingrasaminte organice- protectia calitatii mediului. Editura Ion Ionescu de la Brad Iasi.*

[21] Madejou, E., Lopez, R., Murillo, J., & Cabrera, F. (2001). Agricultural use of three (sugar-but) vinasse composts effect on crops and chemical properties of a Cambisoil soil in the Guadalquivirriver Valleey (SW Spain). *Agriculture, Ecosystems and Enviroment*, 84, Sevilla, Spain.

[22] Marini, L., Scotton, M., Klimek, S., Isselstein, J., & Pericle, A. (2007). Effect of local factors on plant species richness and composition of Alpine meadows. Agriculture ecosystems and environment - , 119(3-4), 281-288.

[23] Metera, E., Sakowski, T., Sloniewski, K., & Romanowicz, B. (2010). Grazing as a tool to maintain biodiversity of grassland-a review. *Animal Science Papers and Reports*, 28(4), 315-334.

[24] Oerlemans, J., von, W. O., Boberfeld, D., & Wolf, . (2007). Impact of long-term nutrient supply on plant species diversity in grassland: an experimental approach on conventionally used pastures. *Journal of applied botany and food quality- angewandte botanik*, 31(2), 151-157.

[25] Peeters, A., Maljean, J. F., Biala, K., & Bouckaert, V. (2004). Les indicateurs de biodiversité pour les prairies: un outil d'évaluation de la durabilité des systèmes d'élevage. *Fourrages*, 178, 217-232.

[26] Rotar, I., Pacurar, F., Garda, N., & Morea, A. (2010a). The management of oligotrophic grasslands and the approach of new improvement methods. *Romania Journal of Grassland and forage crops*, 1, 57-70.

[27] Rotar, I., Pacurar, F., Garda, N., & Morea, A. (2010b). The organic-mineral fertilization of a Festuca rubra L grassland in Apuseni Mountain. *Romania Journal of Grassland and forage crops*, 2, 55-60.

[28] Ryser, J. P., Walther, U., & Flisch, R. (2001). Données de base pour la fumure des grandes cultures et des herbages. *Revue suisse d'Agriculture*, 33(3), 80-86.

[29] Samuil, C., Vintu, V., & Iacob, T. (2007). Influence of mineral and organic fertilization on improving the productivity of permanent grassland from forest steppe in the north-eastern part of Romania. *14st Symposium of the European Grassland Federation*, 146-149.

[30] Samuil, C., Vintu, V., Saghin, G., & Popovici, I. C. (2008). Strategies for Using Organic Fertilizers on Permanent Grasslands in north-eastern Romania. *Cercetări Agronomice în Moldova*, XLI(2), Iaşi, 35-40.

[31] Tilman, D., Wedin, D., & Knops, J. (1996). Productivity and sustainability influenced by biodiversity in grassland ecosystems. *Nature*, 379, 718-720.

[32] Vintu, V., Ionel, A., Samuil, C., Iacob, T., & Trofin, A. (2001). Influenţa subprodusului "vinasse" asupra productivităţii pajiştilor permanente din podişul Central Moldovenesc. *Cercetări Agronomice în Moldova*, 3-4, Edit. "Ion Ionescu de la Brad" Iaşi, 95-100.

[33] Vintu, V., Samuil, C., Iacob, T., Postolache, S., & Popovici, I. C. (2007). The biodiversity and agronomic value of mountain permanent grasslands from the north-eastern part of Romania. Gent Belgia. *14st Symposium of the European Grassland Federation*, 528-531.

[34] Vintu, V., Samuil, C., Sarbu, C., Saghin, G., & Iacob, T. (2008). The influence of grassland management on biodiversity in mountainous region of NE Romania. *Grassland Science in Europe*, 13, 183-185.

[35] Vîntu, V., Ionel, A., Iacob, T., & Samuil, C. (2003). Posibilităţi de îmbunătăţire a pajiştilor permanente prin folosire ca fertilizant a subprodusului vinassa. *Lucrări ştiinţifice, seria Agronomie*, Iaşi.

[36] Weigelt, A., Weisser, W. W., Buchmann, N., & Scherer-Lorenzen, M. (2009). Biodiversity for multifunctional grasslands: equal productivity in high-diversity low-input and low-diversity high-input systems. *Biogeosciences*, 6(8), 1695-1706.

[37] (2011). ***, *Statistic Yearbook of Romania.*

[38] (2011). ***, *Eurostat.*

[39] An analysis of the EU organic sector. (2010). ***, *European Commission Directorate-General for Agriculture and Rural Development.*

[40] Abando, Lourdes Llorens, & Rohnerthielen, Elisabeth. (2007). Statistics in focus. *Agriculture and fisheries*, 67.

Chapter 2

Organic Cereal Seed Quality and Production

Ivana Capouchová, Petr Konvalina, Zdeněk Stehno,
Evženie Prokinová, Dagmar Janovská,
Hana Honsová, Ladislav Bláha and Martin Káš

Additional information is available at the end of the chapter

http://dx.doi.org/10.5772/53073

1. Introduction

At least 1.8 million hectares of main cereal species are under organic management (including in-conversion areas). As some of the world's large cereal producers (such as India, China and the Russian Federation) did not provide land use details, it can be assumed that the area is larger than shown here [1]. Comparing this figure with FAO's figure for the world's harvested cereal area of 384 million hectares [2], 0.5 percent of the total cereal area is under organic management.

Wheat (*Triticum* L.) in general and bread wheat (*Triticum aestivum* L.) in particular, is the most frequent crop in organic farming, the same as in conventional farming. It is grown on a total area of more than 700 000 ha [1]. Bread wheat is the most important crop in the Czech Republic as well. In 2010, it represented almost 25 % of the organic farming land [3]. An organically grown bread wheat provides a low yield rate (3.26 $t.ha^{-1}$) [3]. As for the conventional farming, the yield rate amounts to 5.24 $t.ha^{-1}$ [4]. The organically grown bread wheat yield rate achieves 62 % of the conventionally grown bread wheat. Foreign literary sources often mention the organically grown bread wheat achieving up to 80 % of the yield rate provided by the conventionally grown bread wheat [5].

Oat is one of the most suitable cereal species for organic farming [6]. As it has low requirements on growing conditions, it is a suitable crop for organic farming in Central Europe [7]. There is a relatively wide range of use of oat. Naked oat is a suitable food crop [8]. Common oat is mostly used as a fodder crop [9]. It is the second most frequent crop (just after bread wheat) in the Czech organic farming system. The common oat growing area represents 5,000 hectares and its average yield rate represents 2.5 t/ha [3].

The paragraph above indicates a lower productivity of the organically grown cereal crop stands. A deficiency of certified organic seeds and a serious necessity of an application of own farm saved seed are the factors that might provoke it. For this reason, a question of quality in various provenances of seed is to be answered in this chapter.

2. Legislation of use of seed in organic farming

The Council Regulation (EC) No. 834/2007 of the 28th of June 2007, and the Commission Regulation (EC) No. 889/2008, of the 5th of September 2008, are the most important European legislative instructions addressing organic farming, and are binding for all member states of the European Union. They lay down the law to solely use organic seeds in order to establish organic crop stands. The seed must originate from plants being grown in compliance with the organic farming rules for at least one generation. Seed multiplication is an extremely difficult process. The reproduction crop stand and seed must meet the requirements of the seed certification and authorization procedure as conventional plants and seed do, but organic farming does not allow the use of any pesticides or mineral nitrogenous fertilizers, etc. Organic farmers may use certified organic seeds or farm seed in order to establish the crop stand. They may also apply for an exception (derogation) and use the conventional untreated seed.

2.1. Farm saved seed use

Use of the farm seeds (the seeds produced at a own organic farm) is allowed and any obligatory application for authorization is not required. A farmer should, however, take into account that repeated application of the farm seeds may have a negative effect on the yield rate and health of the crop stand. If the farm seeds of a registered variety are used, a farmer must pay fees to the owner of the breeding rights. Such fees are lower than the standard price for the license (it is even included in the price for the certified organic seeds). The fees (which are usually obligatory but reasonable) for the application of the farm seeds and potato seedlings are not obligatory for small farmers. Moreover, each member state of the European Union has regularized the amount of the fees with legislative regulations.

2.2. Conventional seed use

If there are not any organic seeds available, or left from the previous farming years, seeds coming from the conventional crop stands are allowed. Anyway, the seed needn't be treated with any plant treatment, which are not allowed by the organic farming regulation. An application for an exception to be made,regarding the use of the conventional seeds within the organic farming system, is considered and granted by a public authority (it is usually an accredited organisational unit of the Czech Ministry of Agriculture). The total amount of exceptions tends to be limited, but there is a deficiency of the organic seeds available on the market.

2.3. Information on the availability of the certified organic seeds

Each member state of the European Union is obliged to set up „a database of organic seeds" (Database). A producer or a supplier of the organic seeds is obliged to insert all the varieties into the Database (the variety missing in the Database is considered as an unavailable variety). Before registering the variety (i. e. inserting it into the Database), the farmer has to provide proof at a review he was put under. The control system must comply with the regulations of the European Union. Moreover, the farmer must prove his seeds meet all the legislative requirements for reproductive material. Data inserted into the Database are regularly updated. There is a list of the obligatory items: the scientific name of the species and variety, the supplier's name and contact, the country which the variety has been registered in, the date the seeds have been available from, the amount of seeds, the name and number code of the control institution which has executed the least control and has issued the certificate on the organic seeds and potato seedlings. If the variety is missing in the official Database, an exception can be granted and the conventional seeds are allowed to be applied. Each member state of the European Union has set up its own database. There is a list of the certified organic seeds databases available in EU member states (Table 1).

3. Production of cereal seeds - An example from the Czech Republic

An increasing number of existing organic farms indicates that certified organic farming has been becoming more and more attractive. The number of Czech organic farms amounts to 3,920 and the organic farms cover a total area of 482,927 ha which represents 11.40 % of the whole agricultural land area [4]. Arable land, nevertheless, covers only 12.27 % of the total area (it means 59,281 ha). The above-mentioned data reflect an unsuitable structure of the organic farming. It has arisen from the previous setting of subventional instruments but also the fact that the arable land farming has always been very difficult and required specific knowledge.

The total area of land where the organic cereals are grown amounts to almost 30,000 ha. Bread wheat is the most frequent cereal species grown in accordance with the organic farming principles in the Czech Republic. In 2010, it covered 8,872 ha of the organic land and represented 22 % of all the organically grown cereal species in the Czech Republic [4]. Although it belongs to the most demanding cereal species, it is able to provide an even higher yield rate than the other organically grown cereal species (e. g. bread wheat – 3.26 $t.ha^{-1}$, spelt wheat – 2.91 $t.ha^{-1}$, rye – 2.82 $t.ha^{-1}$, barley – 2.82 $t.ha^{-1}$, oat – 2.54 $t.ha^{-1}$, triticale – 2.95 $t.ha^{-1}$; all the above-mentioned yield rate values were measured in 2010).

3.1. Supply of organic seeds in the Czech Republic

Data concerning the structure of multiplication crop stands, certified seed and the range of seed at the market, were obtained from the Department of seed and planting materials of the Central Institute for Supervising and Testing in Agriculture and the Ministry of Agriculture of the Czech Republic.

Country	Link
Austria	http://www.ages.at
Belgium	http://www.organicxseeds.com
Bulgaria	http://www.organicxseeds.com
Cyprus	http://www.moa.gov.cy
Czech Republic	http://www.ukzuz.cz
Denmark	http://planteapp.dlbr.dk
Estonia	http://www.plant.agri.ee
Finland	http://www.evira.fi
France	http://www.semences-biologiques.org
Germany	http://www.organicxseeds.com
Greece	http://www.minagric.gr
Hungary	http://www.nebih.gov.hu
Ireland	http://www.organicseeds.agriculture.gov.ie
Italy	http://www.ense.it
Latvia	http://www.vaad.gov.lv
Luxembourg	http://www.organicxseeds.com
Netherlands	http://www.biodatabase.nl
Poland	http://ec.europa.eu/agriculture/organic
Portugal	http://www.dgadr.pt
Slovak Republic	http://www.uksup.sk
Slovenia	http://www.arhiv.mkgp.gov.si
Spain	http://www.magrama.gob.es
Sweden	http://www.jordbruksverket.se
United Kingdom	http://www.organicxseeds.com

Table 1. Database of the certified organic seeds registered in each member state of the European Union (data updated within 1st July 2012)

Between 2008/09 and 2010/11 there was a gradual increase in the land area used for organic cereal seed production. Nevertheless, they represented 1.5 % (349 ha) of the total organic land area in 2009 in the Czech Republic. Regarding the average model seeding rate of 220 $kg.ha^{-1}$, we would need 5,008 t of seed to plant the entire area of cereals in a particular year. In 2009, the average grain yield of organic cereals in the Czech Republic represented 2.94 $t.ha^{-1}$[10]. It means we would need a multiplication area of 1,703 ha providing that 100% of the seed were certified as organic seed. In 2009, seed were reproduced on 20.5% of the required land area. It is unrealistic that 100% of grown seed will be certified as organic. A comparison between the allowed multiplication land surface and amounts of allowed winter wheat seed shows that the major part of harvested seed have not been certified as organic seed in 2009 (Table 2). In the same year, 90.95 t of the winter wheat seed were certified as organic. However, this winter wheat was grown on 125 ha of land. It means that the major part of the harvested material did not meet the requirements of the seed certification procedure (same as the major part of the other cereal species). The range of the reproduced organic cereal species is very narrow. The growing of the suitable varieties on the local farm land and under local climatic conditions is strongly limited, because of limited organic seed availability.

Since 2009, organic farmers have asked for permit to use a lot of conventional untreated seed. In 2009, 398 exceptions for 1,664 t of seed were granted (Table 3). Except for the certified organic seed (Table 2) and conventional untreated seed (Table 3), the organic farmers also used their own (saved) seed in order to establish the crop stands. There is not enough information on the applied amount of farm saved seed. Therefore, the following model amount of seeds was used for 2009: amount of certified organic seed = 281 t/seeding rate of 0.22 $t.ha^{-1}$ = 1,277 ha of the seeded surface; amount of conventional untreated seed = 1,664 t/ seeding rate of 0.22 $t.ha^{-1}$ = 7,564 ha of the sown surface. The area of grown cereals represented 22,762 ha - 1,227 ha - 7,564 ha = 13,971 ha where the farm saved seed were used. The share of each seed type is presented in Figure 1.

Species	2008-2009				2009-2010				2010-2011[2]	
	Seed production		Certified seed		Seed production		Certified seed		Seed production	
	NV[1]	ha	NV	t	NV	ha	NV	t	NV	ha
Winter wheat	5	72	4	73	7	125	5	91	4	102
Spring wheat	1	13	1	23	-	-	-	-	1	15
Spelt	2	66	2	159	2	89	2	79	3	143
Spring barley	2	21	1	21	2	26	-		3	20
Triticale	-	-	-	-	1	18	1	8	2	45
Winter rye	-	-	-	-	1	8	1	8	2	37
Naked oat	2	28	2	23	2	34	2	28	1	15
Oat	2	27	-	-	2	50	2	40	2	44
Total	14	**227**	**10**	**299**	**17**	**349**	**13**	**254**	**18**	**422**

Remark: [1]NV = number of varieties; [2]no seed certified

Table 2. Seed production and certified seed offered in the Czech Republic

The use of organic seed becomes more important in many European countries thanks to the legislative measures and increasing demand for the organic products [11]. It is, nevertheless, one of the most developing parts of organic agriculture [12]. However, the total supply of organic seed is still quite low. The high proportion of common farm seed coming from repeated seeding contributes to a reduction of the yield rate of the crop stands [13]. The seed certification process is very demanding, as the organic seed undergo the review of the Central Institute for Supervising and Testing in Agriculture of organic farming [14], but organic farming regulations do not allow the use of any pesticides, etc. [15].

Species	2009		2010	
	Number of exceptions	Seed (t)	Number of exceptions	Seed (t)
Bread wheat	66	271	112	515
Spelt	5	78	9	8
Barley	47	129	77	319
Triticale	86	651	76	455
Rye	23	12	20	42
Oat	161	523	174	444
Total	398	1664	468	1783

Table 3. Exceptions for conventional untreated seed use in the Czech Republic

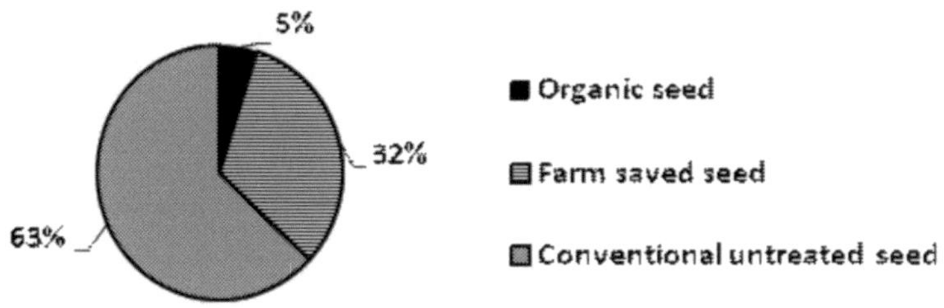

Figure 1. Seed use in organic farming in the Czech Republic (2009) (%)

3.2. Preference and expectations of the Czech organic farmers related to seeds

A questionnaire survey was carried out between 2009 and 2010; 329 questionnaires were sent to organic farmers working on arable land, of which 42% were sent back. The farmers were asked to answer nine questions. The questionnaires were converted into electronic versions and assessed by the contingency tables in the Excel program.

A further part of the questionnaire aimed to find out how organic farmers find and gather information on seeds. The main information resources are as follow: the internet, consultancy, from the Association of Organic Farmers and seed companies. The official database of the certified organic seed (http://www.ukzuz.cz/Folders/2295-1-Ekologicke+osivo.aspx) is also frequently used by the organic farmers (Table 4). The obligation to document the absence of the certified organic seed when applying for a exception in the conventional untreated seed use, is one of the important reasons. Most of the organic farmers (75% of the farms) would prefer the certified organic seed if the supply was sufficient and prices favourable (Table 4). Only 14% of the farms explicitly prefer conventional untreated seed. The suitability of varieties and transport distance are other reasons for the farm saved seed preference (Table 4).

Reason for farm saved seed use (%)		Use of organic seed database (%)		Would you prefer organic seed ? (%)	
Suitability of varieties	16	Yes, I use the database	51	Yes, I would	75
Seed price	37	Yes, I sometimes use	16	No, I would not	14
Transport distance	18	I know but I do not use	20	I do not know	11
Supply	24	I have no access	7		
Others	5	Others	6		

Table 4. Organic farmers' attitudes to seed issues

4. Quality of organic seed – Results of experiments

Data and outcomes being analysed in this chapter have resulted from the trials executed by the authors, and they are described in detail below. They are based on A) results of standard seed laboratory test (biological traits and health), B) results of the field trials.

4.1. Material

Used varieties and seed provenances are described in Table 5. Three categories of seeds were collected in the Czech Republic: the certified organic seeds (O), the conventional untreated seeds (C) and the organic farm seeds (Farm seed I., Farm seed II.). The following cereals species were tested in the research trials and analysed: bread wheat (*Triticum aestivum* L.) – SW Kadrilj variety; two varieties of hulled oat (*Avena sativa* L.) – Neklan and Vok varieties; naked oat (*Avena nuda* L.) –Izak and Saul varieties; and spring barley (*Hordeum vulgare* L.) –Pribina variety.

4.1.1. Methods

Field trials were sown during the experimental years 2010 and 2011 in a randomized, complete block design on organic certified trial field in two locations in Prague (Czech University of Life Sciences Prague; Crop Research Institute in Prague) and in Ceske Budejovice (University of South Bohemia in České Budějovice). The seeding rate was adjusted for a density of 350 germinable grains per m^2. Rows were 125 mm wide. The plots were treated in compliance with European legislation - European Council Regulation (EC) No. 834/2007 and European Commission Regulation (EC) No. 889/2008.

Crop	Cultivar	Seed provenance
Naked oat	Saul	Organic certified (EC), conventional untreated (C), Farm saved seed from better growing conditions (Farm seed I.), Farm saved seed from worse growing conditions (Farm seed II.)
	Izák	
Hulled oat	Vok	
	Neklan	
Bread wheat	SW Kadrilj	
Barley	Pribina	

Table 5. Analysed cultivars and provenances

Characteristics of the trial stations: The Czech University of Life Sciences Prague (50°04 ′N,14°62′E): warm and mid-dry climate, soil type - brown soil, kind of soil - loamy clay soil, altitude of 295 m. The Crop Research Institute in Prague - Ruzyne (50°08′N,14°30′E): warm mid-dry climate, soil type - degraded chernozem, kind of soil - clay and loamy soil, altitude of 340 m. The University of South Bohemia in Ceske Budejovice (48°98′N, 14°45′E): Mild warm climate, soil type – pseudogley cambisols, kind of soil - loamy sand soil, altitude of 388 m.

Analyses of seed contamination with fungi (before seeding and after harvest): The method of isolation of micromycets inside an cultivation media was applied in order to evaluate the rate of grain contamination with microscopic fungi. A universal cultivation media - PDA (Potato Dextrose Agar - HiMedia) was used in the experiment. Incubation lasted from seven to ten days and it was run in a dark room and in a temperature of 20°C. Each sample was repeated five times, there were ten grains included in each repetition. Mixed colonies were cleaned and sorted before the determination, clean isolates of fungi were determined, therefore. The number of isolated colonies was visually determined, the determination of micromycets was executed with microscopes and it was based on the microscopical morphological traits.

Laboratory germination and energy of germination (before seeding and after harvest): 100 caryopses of each sample were used and repeated four times, they were put into plastic bowls with perforated caps, on wet folded filtration paper. The bowls were placed into a ventilated air-conditioned box where 20°C was the inside temperature. The energy of germination was assessed four days later (by counting of usual germinated caryopses). Laboratory germination was assessed by the same procedure eight days later.

Laboratory emergence and energy of emergence (before seeding and after harvest): 100 caryopses of each sample were put in coarse sand, 3 cm deep, four times. A 1 cm wide wet sand layer (characterised by 60% humidity) was placed at the bottom of the bowl. The caryopses were put onto the sand layer; they were slightly pressed and covered with dry sand. The laboratory emergence was determined at the temperature of 15°C. Seven days later, the energy of emergence was assessed, and 14 days later, the laboratory emergence was determined by deduction of the emerged caryopses.

The Statistica 9.0 (StatSoft. Inc., USA) program was used for statistical data analysis. Regression and correlation analyses provided the evaluation of interdependence. The comparison of varieties and their division into statistically different categories were provided by the *Tukey HSD* test.

4.2. Oat (*Avena sativa* L., *Avena sativa* var. *nuda*)

Results of the evaluation of the microscopical fungi occurrence on seeds, found out by isolation and cultivation of colonies on the cultivation media, are shown in Table 6. The seeds were most seriously affected by *Penicillium* spp. colonies. 6.3 colonies per 10 grains – this was the mean number of colonies (*Fusarium* spp., *Alternaria* spp., *Penicillium* spp.) occurring on the seeds before to direct seeding. The hulled oat was more seriously affected than the naked oat. The individual varieties were affected by a similar situation. Neklan was the most seriously affected variety. There were negligible differences between the seed categories (certified organic seeds, conventional untreated seeds, farm seeds originating from organic production) seen from the seed origin point of view. Differences in *Alternaria* spp. occurrence rate between the individual oat species were detected ($P < 0.05$) (*Tukey HSD* test). The common oat caryopses'affection was double to the naked oat caryopses. [16] gives a possible explanation. The microscopical fungi occurrence is stronger on the surface of hulls. The hulled oat is harvested despite the affected hulls, whereas the naked oat caryopses lose their hulls during harvest; therefore, the harvested grains are less contaminated with fungi. Both oat species were characterised by a similar rate of contamination with the other microscopical fungi species (e.g. *Penicillium* spp.). *Rhizopus nigricans* was also detected in most of the samples. Results of the correlation analysis (Table 8) show a strong relationship between the individual biological traits. We have also detected a positive middle correlation between the occurrence of *Alternaria* spp. fungi, germination and emergence rate.

The research was aimed also at the detection of the transmission of fungi micromycets onto the following seed generation. When studying and evaluating the first generation of seed,we found that the seed contamination rate was not influenced by the growing technology applied on the parent seed crop stands (Tables 6 and 7). As for the following seed generation (Tables 9 and 10), it was not significantly influenced by the seed origin – *Tukey HSD* test ($P < 0.05$). As for the following seed generation, a difference in the occurrence rate of *Fusarium* spp. colonies between the oat species has been found out. The hulled oat was more seriously affected because of the harvest of grains covered with the contaminated hulls [16]. There were not any significant correlations between the microscopical fungi contamination rate and the biological traits of seeds (Table 11).

The influence of seed health conditions on an expansion of diseases throughout the growing period has not yet been ascertained. No varieties or localities were affected by any diseases being caused by the pathogens we had determined on the seeds. They were not affected by any other pathogens being trasmitted by seeds either. The total rate of contamination of the caryopses with microscopical fungi was influenced by weather conditions during vegetation period. The year of 2010 had been wetter, which caused a higher rate of grain contamination. The hulled oat was more seriously contaminated than the naked oat; it was caused by a fact that the hulled oat caryopses get less dry, that makes ideal conditions for an expansion of the fungi pathogens [16]. The strong rate of caryopses' contamination with *Penicillium* spp. colonies was surprising, as these fungi are considered as waste disposal pathogens.

Factor		***Fusarium* spp.** (no. colonies/10 grains)	***Alternaria spp. (no. colonies/10 grains)***	***Penicillium spp. (no. colonies/10 grains)***
Oat	Hulled	0.7±0.6^{a}	2.0±0.7^{b}	4.3±2.4^{a}
	Naked	0.4±0.3^{a}	1.1±0.7^{a}	4.1±3.4^{a}
Variety	Izak	0.5±0.4^{a}	1.1±0.7^{a}	3.7±2.2^{a}
	Saul	0.3±0.2^{a}	1.2±0.8^{a}	4.5±4.5^{a}
	Vok	0.5±0.6^{a}	2.0±1.0^{a}	2.9±1.4^{a}
	Neklan	0.8±0.6^{a}	2.0±0.3^{a}	5.7±2.4^{a}
Seed	Organic	0.5±0.6^{a}	1.7±1.1^{a}	4.8±3.6^{a}
	Conventional	0.6±0.5^{a}	1.6±0.8^{a}	4.1±2.0^{a}
	Farm saved seed	0.5±0.4^{a}	1.4±0.6^{a}	3.7±3.2^{a}
Year	2010	0.3±0.5^{a}	2.0±0.7^{a}	5.1±3.3^{b}
	2011	0.8±0.4^{b}	1.2±0.8^{b}	3.3±2.2^{a}
Total		0.5±0.5	1.6±0.8	4.2±2.9

Remark: Different letters show the statistical differences in *Tukey HSD* test between varieties, $P < 0.05$;

Table 6. Contamination of seed by microscopic fungi colonies - seed before seeding (mean + SD)

Our research has not ascertained any transmission of micromycets or pathogens onto the emerged plants or the following seed generation either. Such a finding is, nevertheless, relevant to oat which is extensive [17] and less bred than the other cereal species. The contamination of seeds with *Penicillium* spp. colonies usually leads to a reduction of germination and emergence. The contamination of caryopses with *Fusarium* spp. colonies did not cause any serious reduction of germination or emergence during the trials. The Czech legal notice on the marketing of cereal seeds (Regulation No. 369/2009), based on the European Union legislation, does not stipulate any limits of the rate of occurrence of *Fusarium* for oat grains. As for the other cereal species, the limit of 10 % has been set by law. We have based our research on the fact that the same limit may be accepted by oat too. Concerning the health conditions of seeds, the occurrence of *Fusarium* spp. was one of the studied and evaluated pathogens. The detected amount of *Fusarium* spp. did not have any negative effect on the seeds. The experiment has also shown that the rate of contamination with *Fusarium* did not reach the limit of 10 percent in the organic farming system in 2011 either. However, the year of 2011 was characterised by a high precipitation rate in June and July, which played a positive role for *Fusarium* expansion within spikes. The average rate of contamination of the naked oat grains with *Fusarium* reached 1.3 percent in 2011, whereas it reached 8.3 percent within the common oat grains the same year. Therefore, it is highly recommended to use own farm saved seed in order to establish a crop stand if there is a deficiency of the certified organic seeds. We have to take the rate of occurrence of *Penicillium* spp. into account. However, the proper farm seeds must come from the crop stands being grown in accordance with the principles of rmultiplication agrotechnology. According to [14], such principles include a good-quality cropping, a parcel rid of post-harvest residues, ideal land-climatic conditions, a careful harvest, etc.

Factor	Parameter	Energy of Germination (%)	Germination (%)	Energy of Emergence (%)	Emergence (%)
Oat	Hulled	77±24[a]	85±13[a]	69±12[a]	78±11[a]
	Naked	78±28[a]	82±25[a]	65±28[a]	71±28[a]
Variety	Izak	93±7[a]	96±2[a]	84±4[b]	87±3[b]
	Saul	63±33[a]	68±29[a]	46±30[a]	55±3[a]
	Vok	69±30[a]	81±16[a]	65±12[ab]	73±13[ab]
	Neklan	85±14[a]	90±8[a]	74±10[ab]	82±8[ab]
Seed	Organic	75±30[a]	84±18[a]	67±21[a]	74±21[a]
	Conventional	86±25[a]	88±23[a]	73±25[a]	79±24[a]
	Farm seed	71±21[a]	79±17[a]	62±19[a]	70±18[a]
Year	2010	92±8[a]	93±7[a]	73±7[a]	82±6[a]
	2011	63±29[b]	75±23[b]	61±28[a]	66±27[a]
Total		78±25	84±19	67±21	74±21

Remark: Different letters show the statistical differences in *Tukey HSD* test between varieties, $P < 0.05$;

Table 7. Biological traits - seed before seeding (mean + SD)

Parameter		Mean+SD	1	2	3	4	5	6
Fusarium spp.	1	0.5±0.5						
Alternaria spp.	2	1.6±0.9	-0.23[ns]					
Penicillium spp.	3	4.2±2.9	-0.10[ns]	0.32[ns]				
EG[1](%)	4	78±25	-0.24[ns]	0.44*	0.33[ns]			
Germination(%)	5	84±19	-0.10[ns]	0.42*	0.33[ns]	0.93**		
EE[2](%)	6	67±21	0.07[ns]	0.29[ns]	0.35[ns]	0.83**	0.95**	
Emergence(%)		74±21	0.04[ns]	0.41*	0.36[ns]	0.86**	0.97**	0.98**

Remark: *$P < 0.05$; **$P < 0.01$; [ns] not significant; [1]EG = energy of germination; [2]EE = energy of emergence

Table 8. Results of the correlation analysis (seed before seeding)

Factor		*Fusarium spp. (no. colonies/10 grains)*	*Alternaria spp. (no. colonies/10 grains)*	*Penicilium spp. (no.colonies/10 grains)*
Oat	Hulled	1.4±0.8^{b}	4.6±2.2^{b}	2.9±2.4^{a}
	Naked	0.7±0.7^{a}	2.4±1.8^{a}	4.3±2.9^{b}
Variety	Izak	0.8±0.5^{ab}	2.4±1.5^{a}	4.2±2.1^{a}
	Saul	0.6±0.9^{b}	2.4±2.4^{a}	2.3±3.0^{a}
	Vok	1.4±0.8^{a}	4.9±2.0^{b}	2.6±3.6^{a}
	Neklan	1.3±0.8^{a}	4.4±2.1^{b}	3.3±1.8^{a}
Seed	Organic	1.0±0.7^{a}	3.5±2.6^{a}	3.6±2.8^{a}
	Conventional	1.2±0.7^{a}	3.4±2.3^{a}	3.9±2.9^{a}
	Farm saved seed	0.9±1.0^{a}	3.7±2.0^{a}	3.3±2.6^{a}
Year	2010	1.2±0.9^{a}	3.2±2.7^{a}	3.7±3.3^{a}
	2011	1.0±0.8^{a}	3.8±1.8^{a}	3.5±2.1^{a}
Locality	CULS	1.5±1.0^{a}	3.2±2.4^{a}	4.3±2.9^{a}
	USB	0.9±0.7^{a}	3.7±2.6^{a}	4.2±3.0^{a}
	CRI	0.7±0.5^{a}	3.6±1.9^{a}	2.3±1.8^{a}
Total		1.1±0.8	3.5±2.3	3.6±2.7

Remark: Different letters show the statistical differences in *Tukey HSD* test between varieties, $P < 0.05$;

Table 9. Contamination of seed by microscopical fungi colonies - harvested seed (mean + SD)

Factor		Energy of Germination (%)	Germination (%)	Energy of Emergence (%)	Emergence (%)
Oat	Hulled	88±17^{a}	90±16^{a}	78±14^{a}	84±13^{a}
	Naked	92±5^{a}	93±4^{a}	78±11^{a}	85±8^{a}
Variety	Izak	93±4^{a}	95±3^{a}	81±8^{a}	88±4^{a}
	Saul	90±13^{a}	92±10^{a}	75±13^{a}	83±12^{a}
	Vok	84±5^{a}	87±4^{a}	76±13^{a}	82±10^{a}
	Neklan	92±20^{a}	94±20^{a}	81±15^{a}	87±15^{a}
Seed	Organic	90±12^{a}	93±9^{a}	79±12^{a}	86±10^{a}
	Conv.	89±8^{a}	91±7^{a}	76±5^{a}	84±5^{a}
	Farm	90±16^{a}	92±16^{a}	78±17^{a}	85±16^{a}
Year	2010	93±4^{b}	95±3^{b}	77±7^{a}	86±7^{a}
	2011	87±16^{a}	89±15^{a}	79±16^{a}	84±14^{a}
Locality	CULS	91±4^{a}	93±4^{a}	80±9^{a}	86±8^{a}
	USB	94±4^{a}	95±3^{a}	82±7^{a}	87±4^{a}
	CRI	85±20^{a}	87±18^{a}	73±17^{a}	82±17^{a}
Total		90±12	92±11	78±12	85±11

Remark: Different letters show the statistical differences in *Tukey HSD* test between varieties, $P < 0.05$;

Table 10. Biological traits of seed - harvested seed (mean + SD)

http://dx.doi.org/10.5772/53073

Parameter		Mean + SD	1	2	3	4	5	6
Fusarium spp.	1	1.1±0,8						
Alternaria spp.	2	3.5±2,3	0.47**					
Penicilium spp.	3	3.6±2,7	-0.05^{ns}	-0.16^{ns}				
EG[1] (%)	4	90±12	0.03^{ns}	-0.04^{ns}	-0.01^{ns}			
Germination (%)	5	92±11	0.06^{ns}	-0.04^{ns}	-0.01^{ns}	0.99**		
EE[2] (%)	6	78±12	0.03^{ns}	0.07^{ns}	-0.11^{ns}	0.74**	0.72**	
Emergence (%)		85±11	0.01^{ns}	0.01^{ns}	-0.12^{ns}	0.84**	0.83**	0.93**

Remark: $^{*}P <0.05$; $^{**}P <0.01$; ^{ns} not significant;[1]EG = energy of germination;[2]EE = energy of emergence

Table 11. Results of the correlation analysis (harvested seed)

4.3. Bread wheat (*Triticum aestivum* L.)

The spring wheat cultivar SW Kadrilj registered in the Czech Republic has been selected as a model variety. The experiments aimed at the evaluation of selected diseases and seed quality were organised in 3 localities for 2 years (2010 and 2011). Experimental plots in particular localities were sown with seeds of different origin (organic certified, farm saved seed and conventional untreated) whose health state and quality is described in Tables 12 and 13.

Factor		*Fusarium spp. (no. colonies/10 grains)*	*Alternaria spp. (no. colonies/10 grains)*
Year	2010	1.4±1.1^{a}	2.0±1.0^{a}
	2011	0.1±0.2^{a}	0.7±1.3^{a}
Seed origin	Organic	0.7±1.0^{a}	0.5±0.7^{a}
	Conventional	0.2±0.3^{a}	1.0±1.4^{a}
	Farm saved seed	1.5±1.5^{a}	2.6±0.5^{a}
Total		0.8±1.0	1.4±1.0

Table 12. Contamination of seed with *Fusarium* spp. and *Alternaria* spp. (seed before seeding)

Factor		Energy of Germination (%)	Germination (%)	Energy of Emergence (%)	Emergence (%)
Year	2010	98±1^{a}	98±1^{a}	78±2^{a}	79±1^{a}
	2011	82±25^{a}	86±20^{a}	68±32^{a}	74±26^{a}
Seed origin	Organic	98±2^{a}	98±2^{a}	83±5^{a}	83±5^{a}
	Conventional	76±32^{a}	81±26^{a}	54±31^{a}	61±24^{a}
	Farm seed	96±1^{a}	97±0^{a}	82±7^{a}	85±7^{a}
Total		90±18	92±15	73±21	77±17

Table 13. Biological traits (seed before seeding)

Infestation of the seed used for seeding with *Fusarium* spp. and *Alternaria* spp. depended on seed provenance. The farm seed was more infested in both years (Table 12). On the other hand seed quality parameters were very similar in categories of seed origin in 2010 but in 2011 the conventional seed had very low seed quality growing to bad conditions during harvest.

In grain after the harvest of experimental plots, there were determined the same parameters as in the initial seed and the obtained data were statisicaly evaluated (Tables 13 and 14).

Factor		***Fusarium* spp. (no. colonies/10 grains)**	***Alternaria* spp. (no. colonies/10 grains)**
Locality	CRI	0.4±0.4[a]	4.3±0.8[a]
	USB	0.9±0.7[a]	4.9±1.5[a]
	CULS	0.8±0,6[a]	5.6±1.8[a]
Year	2010	0.8±0.7[a]	4.9±1.9[a]
	2011	0.6±0.4[a]	5.0±0.9[a]
Seed origin	Organic	0.6±0.7[a]	5.2±1.7[a]
	Conv.	0.9±0.5[a]	4.6±1.9[a]
	Farm	1.0±0.4[a]	5.1±0.8[a]
Total		0.7±0.6	4.9±1.5

Remark: Different letters show the statistical differences in *Tukey HSD* test among parameters within categories. $P < 0.05$;

Table 14. Contamination of seed by microscopical fungi colonies - harvested seed (mean + SD)

Variability within particular categories (locality, year and seed origin) was relatively high. Consequently, no significant differences within the categories were identified (Table 15). Nevertheless, we can observe that in grain harvested from plots sown with farm saved seed, the infestation with *Fusarium* spp. was higher than in the other two categories (Table 15).

In 2010 there was evaluated in addition to *Fusarium* spp. and *Alternaria* spp. also the occurrence of *Cladosporium* spp. that widely infested seed in that year. Micromycets of all three species appeared on seed used for seeding in very similar quantities (Figure 2). *Fusarium* spp. contaminated harvested grain lightly. A higher occurrence has been observed in the case of *Alternaria* spp., *Cladosporium* spp. was prevailing in the CRI localilty.

A similar situation as in 2010 was observed in 2011, mainly as it concerns *Fusarium* spp. (Figure 3). Instead of *Cladosporium* spp. the *Penicilium* spp. was prevailing at that year because it contaminated harvested seed relatively strongly.

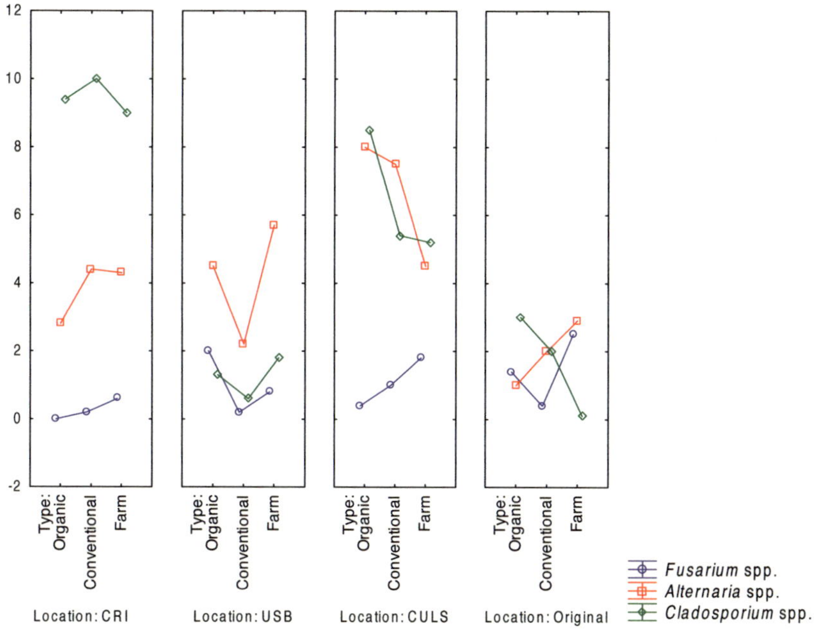

Figure 2. Comparison of infestation in harvested seed of different provenance in 2010 (no.of colonies/10 grains)

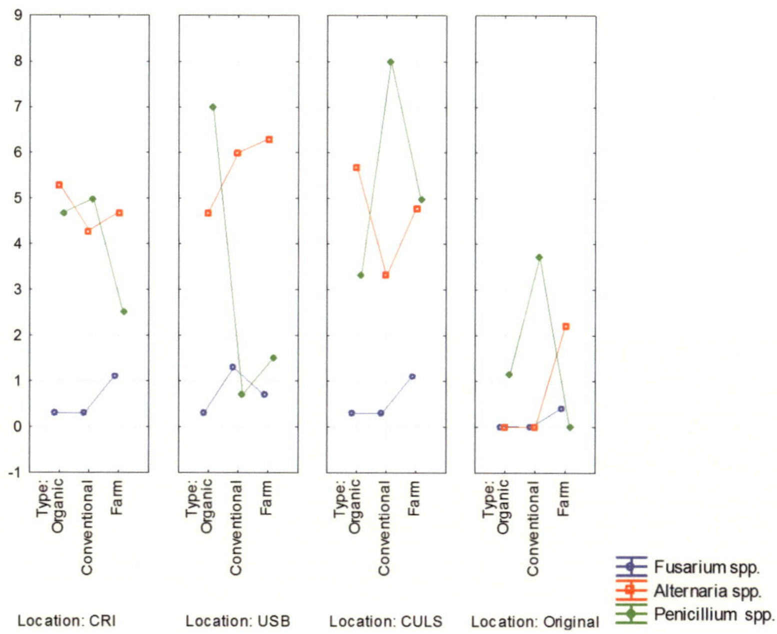

Figure 3. Comparison of infestation in harvested seed of different provenance in 2011

Factor		Energy of Germina-tion (%)	Germina-tion (%)	Energy of Emergence (%)	Emergence (%)	Yield (t.ha^{-1})
Location	CRI	95±5a	97±3^a	82±7^a	88±4^a	2.8±0.6^a
	CULS	97±1^b	99±1^b	85±11^a	89±7^a	5.8±0.7^b
Year	2010	99±0^b	100±0^b	77±8^a	85±5^a	3.8±1.6^a
	2011	94±4^a	96±2^a	89±5^b	92±2^b	4.8±1.9^b
Seed origin	Organic	97±4^a	98±2^a	77±13^a	87±8^a	4.3±2.0^a
	Conventional	97±4^a	98±3^a	84±6^a	88±5^a	4.2±1.9^a
	Farm saved seed	97±5^a	98±3^a	88±4^a	91±2^a	4.4±1.8^a
Total		97±4	98±2	83±9	89±5	4.3±1.7

Remark: Different letters show the statistical differences in *Tukey HSD* testbetween varieties. $P < 0.05$;

Table 15. Biological traits - harvested seed (mean + SD)

Differences among localities in seed quality parameters were not significant. Nevertheless, higher seed quality was determined in seed from CULS – locality Prague – Uhříněves. In general, final values (germination and emergence) were higher than the energy of germination and energy of emergence, respectively. Different conditions during the vegetation period in 2010 and 2011 caused significant differences between the years. Higher germination and energy of germination was not manifested in higher energy of laboratory tested energy of emergence and emergence. Different origin of seed did not influence significantly seed quality parameters.

4.4. Barley (*Hordeum vulgare* L.)

The spring barley variety Xanadu registered in the Czech Republic has been selected as a model variety. As in the case of spring wheat, the experiments aimed at the evaluation of the most important diseases and seed quality were organised in 2 experimental localities (Crop Research Institute Prague – CRI and Czech University of Life Sciences Prague – CULS) for 2 years (2010 and 2011). Experimental plots in both of the localities were sown with seed of different origin (organic certified, organic farm farm saved and conventional untreated) whose health and quality is described in Tables 16 and 17.

Infestation of barley seed used for seeding with *Fusarium* spp. depended more on the year than on seed provenance. Differences between the individual seed provenances were minimal. On the other hand, infestation of barley seed used for seeding with *Alternaria* spp. depended particularly on seed provenance – farm saved seed was more infested in both years. Infestation of the seed with *Penicillium* spp. was affected more by year (Table 16). The quality of the seed used for seeding depended more on the year – values of all the evaluated parameters in 2011 were lower and worse in comparison with the year 2010. The effect of the seed provenance on evaluated seed quality parameters was minimal.

Factor		*Fusarium spp. (no. colonies/10 grains)*	*Alternaria spp. (no. colonies/10 grains)*	*Penicillium spp. (no. colonies/10 grains)*
Year	2010	0.7±0.1[a]	0.6±0.4[a]	1.9±0.6[a]
	2011	0.1±0.1[a]	0.8±1.4[a]	0.2±0.2[b]
Seed origin	Organic	0.4±0.4[a]	0.2±0.3[a]	1.4±1.8[a]
	Conventional	0.4±0.6[a]	0.2±0.3[a]	1.1±0.8[a]
	Farm saved seed	0.4±0.3[a]	1.7±1.0[a]	0.8±0.9[a]
Total		0.4±0.3	0.7±0.9	1.1±1.0

Table 16. Contamination of seed by microscopical fungi (seed before seeding)

Factor		Energy of Germination (%)	Germination (%)	Energy of Emergence (%)	Emergence (%)
Year	2010	99±1[a]	99±1[a]	82±3[a]	87±2[a]
	2011	68±3[b]	89±3[a]	70±2[a]	76±3[a]
Seed origin	Organic	85±20[a]	96±5[a]	76±5[a]	82±4[a]
	Conventional	84±22[a]	93±8[a]	77±8[a]	81±11[a]
	Farm saved seed	81±23[a]	92±8[a]	76±10[a]	81±9[a]
Total		83±16	94±6	76±7	81±6

Table 17. Biological traits (seed before seeding)

In grain, harvested on both of the experimental localities, there were determined the same parameters as in seeds used for seeding. Obtained data are given in Tables 18 and 19 and in Figure 4. Variability within particular categories (locality, year and seed origin) was not high in *Fusarium* spp. infestation of harvested grain (in 2011 was higher, but the differences between both years were not significant). In the case of *Alternaria* spp., there was observed a relatively high (but not significant) difference between both years, and a significant difference between both localities. Differences between the seed origins were relatively small and insignificant. In *Penicillium* spp. infestation of harvested grain was relatively high, statistically significant difference between both years was observed; statistically significant difference between both localities was also observed. On the other hand, the effect of the seed origin was lower (Table 18).

It is evident from the comparison of fungal infestation in harvested seed and seed used for seeding of different provenance (Figure 4), infestation of barley seed used for seeding with

Fusarium spp., *Alternaria* spp. and *Penicillium* spp. was in general lower than infestation of harvested seed on both localities.

Factor		***Fusarium spp. (no. colonies/10 grains)***	***Alternaria spp. (no. colonies/10 grains)***	***Penicillium spp. (no. colonies/10 grains)***
Year	2010	0.4±0.6a	5.1±2.7^a	2.2±1.7^a
	2011	1.3±0.9^a	2.7±2.1^a	6.2±2.0^b
Location	CULS	0.9±1.1^a	2.2±2.4^a	5.5±2.8^b
	CRI	0.8±0.6^a	5.5±1.8^b	2.8±2.1^a
Seed origin	Organic	0.7±0.8^a	3.7±2.5^a	4.2±3.6^a
	Conventional	0.9±0.6^a	3.6±3.9^a	3.6±3.3^a
	Farm seed	1.1±1.2^a	4.4±2.0^a	4.7±1.6^a
Total		0.9±0.8	3.9±2.6	4.2±2.7

Table 18. Contamination of seed by microscopical fungi - harvested seed (mean + SD)

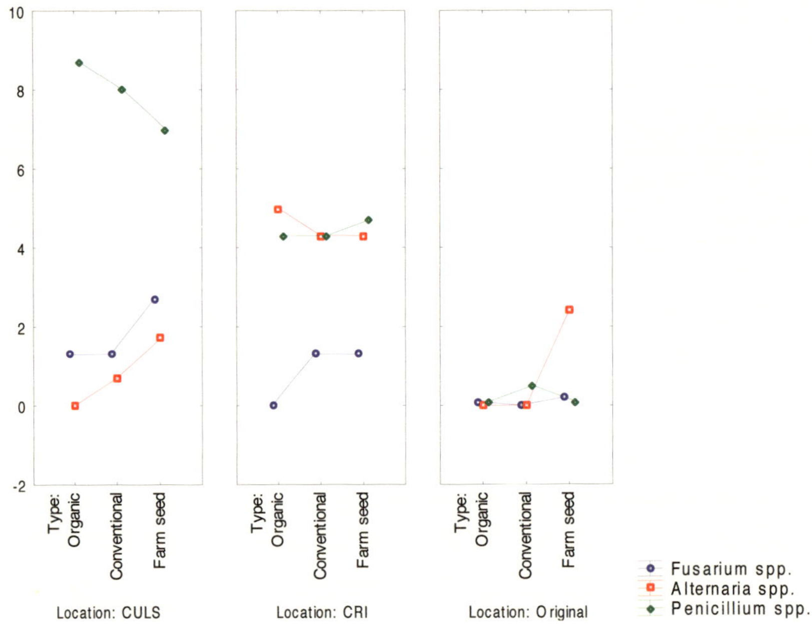

Figure 4. Comparison of infestation in harvested seed of different provenance

Results of quality evaluation of harvested seed are given in Table 18. It is evident from these results, that the effect of locality and year on values of all of evaluated seed quality parameters was higher than the effect of the seed origin. The same situation was observed in the yield of harvested grain – effect of year and locality was relatively high and statistically significant, effect of the seed origin on yield of harvested grain was low.

Factor		Energy of Germination (%)	Germination (%)	Energy of Emergence (%)	Emergence (%)	Yield ($t.ha^{-1}$)
Location	CULS	81±6[a]	87±3[a]	73±10[a]	77±7[a]	6.0±0.4[b]
	CRI	92±3[b]	94±2[b]	77±14[a]	83±10[a]	3.0±1.1[a]
Year	2010	87±10[a]	92±4[a]	66±9[a]	74±6[a]	3.9±2.2[a]
	2011	86±5[a]	89±5[a]	83±7[b]	86±7[b]	5.0±1.2[b]
Origin	Organic	84±12[a]	90±6[a]	74±14[a]	80±10[a]	4.4±1.4[a]
	Conv.	88±4[a]	91±4[a]	79±12[a]	83±8[a]	4.5±2.1[a]
	Farm	88±5[a]	91±5[a]	71±12[a]	78±10[a]	4.5±2.2[a]
Total		86±7	90±4	75±12	80±9	4.5±1.7

Remark: Different letters show the statistical differences in *Tukey HSD* test between varieties. $P < 0.05$;

Table 19. Biological traits of seed - harvested seed (mean + SD)

5. Conclusion

The organic farming has been developing very fast worldwide. There has been, nevertheless, a serious deficiency of certified organic seeds of most of the crops in most of the countries. It also concerns the cereals belonging to the most frequent crops being grown on the organic farms.

There has been the longtime deficiency of the certified organic seeds in the Czech Republic too. The parcels intended for multiplication of seeds cover an insufficient area. Most of the seeds have not been certified because they are highly infected with the diseases transmitted by the seeds themselves. Strict norms for the organic seed certification process should be changed in the near future. Nowadays, the same norms are valid in the organic and conventional farming but any supportive instruments being applied by the conventional farming system are not permitted by the organic farming system (e. g. mineral fertilizers, pesticides, etc.).

The own farm saved seed or the conventional untreated seeds are usually used in order to establish the crop stand because there is a serious deficiency of certified organic seeds. However, the application of conventional untreated seeds does not comply with the organic farming principles. Therefore, the European Union currently started putting permanent pressure on the conventional untreated seeds to be limited. Therefore, if the deficiency of organic seeds persists, a percentage of the applied uncontrolled own farm saved seed is to increase.

Our trials aimed at the evaluation of the influence the seed provenance (the certified organic seeds, the conventional untreated seeds, the farm saved seed) had on the seed parameters and health. Four spring forms of cereals were tested (hulled and naked oat, bread wheat, and barley). The influence of the various seed provenance on the crop stand quality was particularly studied. Moreover, a possible effect of the various seed provenance on seed parameters and health of the following seed generation were also evaluated.

Study of the influence of biological characteristics on the following seed generation has shown that all the seed categories achieve a good-quality level. The seeds originating from certified organic seeds have the best biological characteristics of all. The oat seeds coming from the own farm saved seed had also good qualitative parameters. We have come to similar findings as for the health state of the crop stand. There is not any correlation between the intensity of seed infestation with pathogens and the health state of the following seed generation.

If the laws get more strict, or the conventional untreated seeds are absolutely forbidden by the organic farming system, the deficiency of the certified organic seeds will have to be compensated by the own farm saved seed supply. Anyway, the farm seeds must be reproduced on the parcels having good qualitative parameters and careful agrotechnological methods will be indispensable.

Acknowledgements

Supported by the Ministry of Agriculture of the Czech Republic – NAZV, Grant No. QI 91C123.

Author details

Ivana Capouchová[1], Petr Konvalina[2], Zdeněk Stehno[3], Evženie Prokinová[1], Dagmar Janovská[3], Hana Honsová[1], Ladislav Bláha[3] and Martin Káš[3]

1 Czech University of Life Sciences in Prague, Praha 6-Suchdol, Czech Republic

2 University of South Bohemia in České Budějovice, Č. Budějovice, Czech Republic

3 Crop Research Institute in Prague, Praha 6-Ruzyně, Czech Republic

References

[1] Willer H, Kilcher L., editors. The World of Organic Agriculture. Statistics and Emerging Trends 2009. Bonn and Frick: IFOAM and FiBL; 2009, 309 p.

[2] FAOSTAT: http://faostat.fao.org/ (accesed 15 June 2011).

[3] Hrabalová A. Ročenka ekologického zemědělství v České republice 2010 (Czech Organic Yearbook 2010). Brno: ÚKZÚZ. 2011, 46 p.

[4] MZe. Situační a výhledovázprávaobiloviny 2009 (Cereals yearbook 2009). Praha: MZe, 2009;104 p.

[5] Ingver A, Tamm I, Tamm Ü. Effect of organic and conventional production on yield and the quality of spring cereals. Agronomijas Vēstis (Latvian Journal of Agronomy) 2008;11: 61-67.

[6] Lockeretz W, Shearer G, Kohl DH. Organic Farming in the Corn Belt. Science 1981;211: 540-547.

[7] Leistrumaitė A, Liatukas Ž, Razbadauskienė K. The spring cereal traits of soil cover, disease resistance and yielding essential for organic growing. Agronomy Research 2009;7: 374-380.

[8] Batalova GA, Changzhong R, Rusakova II, Krotova NV. Breeding of naked oats. Russian Agricultural Sciences 2010; 36: 93-95.

[9] Stevens EJ, Armstrong KW,Bezar HJ, GriffinWB, Hampton JB. Fodder Oats: an overview. In: Suttie JM, Reynolds SG. (eds.) Fodder Oats: A World Overview, Plant Production and Protection Series. Rome: FAO; 2004.pp. 11–18.

[10] MZe. Ročenka ekologické zemědělství 2009 (Czech organic yearbook 2009). Praha: MZe ČR, 2009, 44 p.

[11] Václavík, T. (2008): Ročenka českýtrh s biopotravinami. Green marketing, Praha, 65 p.

[12] Shamash J. Developments in seed production. Horticulture Week 2008;41: 2.

[13] Lammerts van Bueren ET, Struik PC, Tiemens-Hulscher M, Jacobsen NE. Concepts of intrinsic value and integrity of plants in organic plant breeding and propagation. Crop Sciences 2003; 43: 1922-1929.

[14] Houba M, Hosnedl V. Osivo a sadba (Seed and Seedlings). Prague: Profi Press. 2002, 186 p.

[15] Lampkin N. Organic farming. Ipswich:Farming press, 1990, 701 p.

[16] Adler A, Lew H, Moudrý J, Štěrba Z, Vrátilová K, Edinger W, Brodacz W, Kiendler E. Microbiological and mycotoxicological quality parameters of naked and covered oats with regard to the production of bran and flakes. Die Bodenkultur 2003; 54: 41-48.

[17] Pszczółkowska A, Fordoński G, Olszewski J, Kulik T, Konopka I. Productivity and seed health of husked oats (*Avena sativa*L.) grown under different soil moisture conditions. Acta Agrobotanica 2010; 63: 127-133.

Chapter 3

Option Models Application of Investments in Organic Agriculture

Karmen Pažek and Črtomir Rozman

Additional information is available at the end of the chapter

http://dx.doi.org/10.5772/52008

1. Introduction

Farmers constantly face decisions about whether to invest in a new production method with increased risks and uncertainties or to maintain the current system without new risks and uncertainties. The possible method to evaluate a new business or investment opportunity is to use traditional discounted cash flow methods [23, 24]. Investment assessment is the very important part of the capital operations and important perception for the success of investment projects. Although the Net Present Value (NPV_t) methodology is widely used by project decision making process, a disadvantage of the NPV_t is that the method does not include the flexibility or uncertainty. Several researchers argue that Net Present Value (NPV_t) is not adequate under uncertain conditions and typically considers projects to be irreversible [1, 4, 8, 29]. To evaluate suitable investment possibilities, an investor-farmer needs to take into account the value of keeping options open, including the impact of sources of uncertainty and risk attitudes. The risk and uncertainty associated with management decisions are included in the formulation of real options problems [8, 30] and real option models [3]. However, real options approach (ROA) rise from the doubt of NPV_t method and can make up for it in assessment investment agricultural projects.

There are some limitations of NPV_t by evaluating agricultural investment project. [32] presented some of them; $NPV_t$is not flexible and only uses information available at the time of the decision. It does not account for changes to the project after the initial decision being made. Further, NPV_t method only emphasize that a prospective project must be positive value. The traditional discount cash will not recommend embedding an option to expansion which is expected to be negative – the expansion is an option and not an obligation. In fact, not all agricultural venture capital projects could make a profit immediately, because the sustainable development needs to be considered. For example, if the agricultural project of seed – improvement, as a long-term project, succeeds, it will greatly improve the food production and increase farmer's income. Real options approach can make up for the deficiencies of $NPV_{t,}$ which greatly enhance the accuracy of investment decisions.

A real option is defined as the value of being able to choose some characteristic of a decision with irreversible consequences, which affects especially on a financial income. Real options uses a flexible approach to uncertainty (i.e. ecological and technological production possibilities, economic efficiency of production, market and trade opportunity) by identifying its sources, developing future business alternatives, and constructing decision rules. It attempts to reduce risk by monitoring the implementation of its decisions and requiring decision making to be adaptive throughout the life cycle of a project.

Further, ROA approach focus on irreversibility of investment in agricultural venture capital project. NPV_t method has such a hypothesis that the investment is reversible, and the investment can not be delayed. In reality, the majority of investment projects are irreversible. This is one of the major theoretical flaws of NPV_tmethod. Real options approach reputes that, in most cases, although the investment is irreversible, investment could be postponed. Many uncertainties in the environment may eventually be eliminated. NPV_t method ignores the strategic value of the projects, such as the opportunity to expand into a new market, to develop natural resources or technology. By taking this method, decision maker will have to consider questions from the static view, and think that the cash flow of investment is fixed, only make decision whether to accept the investments immediately or not. On the contrary, ROA carries on the decision making from dynamic view. What ROA obtains is the expansion of $NPV_,$ which include traditional NPV_t and the value of options [32].

ROA approach takes into consideration the flexibility of agricultural venture capital project. Example, NPV method does not allow for the management flexibility that is often present. Many investments opportunities have options embedded in them and the traditional NPV misses this extra value because it treats investors as passive. However, by using ROA, decision maker can adjust value by reacting to changing conditions. For example, they could expand operations of the project if the outlook seems attractive, while reduce the scope of activities if the future outlook is unattractive. When considering uncertainty and managerial flexibility, NPV does not properly capture the non-linear nature of the cash flow distribution or the changing risk profile over time. In fact, the agricultural reproduction process is the process that the social economy reproduction and the nature reproduction are interwoven, so the benefit of agricultural project has the big instability. ROA takes into consideration the flexibility of agricultural investment project, which confirms to the characteristic of agriculture capita project evaluation [32].

Theoretical advances in real options methodology have been formulated and assimilated in several empirical applications [7, 20, 21]. The practice of real options approach has played a positive role in reachening the theory of real options. Therefore real options, just as the same as financial options, is not only the right to investment, but also gradually become a kind of investment philosophy. Real options theory is increasingly used in industry projects too.

Real options methodology was used to evaluate organic agriculture [31]. The authors stressed the new European policy measures, where adoption of environmental friendly production systems should be considered. The adoptions is includes risk and uncertainty and to overcome this parameters well designed policy schemes are required. The study attempts to examine the effects of income variability upon the decision on adopting or not environmental friendly production systems in order to evaluate the organic financial incentives to farmers by introducing the real options methodology. The technology adoption of a free-stall dairy housing under irreversibility and uncertainty and its implications in the design of environmental policies was examined [26]. Further, the stochastic dynamic model of investment decision of an individual farmer under risk in the presence of irreversibility and technical change was assessed [9]. [18] explore the potential of the real options approach for analysing farmers' choice to switch from conventional to organic farming. The model for effect-assessment of prices variability by the decision to invest in conservation with application to terrace construction was developed too [33]. A model for determining optimal entry and exit thresholds for investment in irrigation systems when there is given irreversibility and uncertain returns with price and yield as stochastic variables were developed [25]. The model for investment decision to convert farmland to urban as an irreversible investment under uncertainty when use of this land is restricted by government policies so as to protect the environment were developed [29]. The appliance of real options evaluation is showed on model of plum and plum brandy as an extension. The research implies that plum plantation has an option value (call value) regarding extension to plum brandy production. This option was determined using the most frequently used option valuation method - Black-Scholes model [10]. The impact of price uncertainty and expectations of declining fixed costs on the optimal timing site specific crop management was presented by [11]. However, there are presentedsome more studies on the application of real options in agriculture [13, 15, 16, 17, 19, 22].

In the presented research the use of the decision making process and its tools for evaluating investments in organic spelt processing business alternatives using elements of the real options methodology is presented. The study focuses on the impact of Net Present Value (NPV_t) as a parameter for investment decisions in the framework of Cost Benefit Analysis (CBA) and the real options model (Black-Scholes and binominal model).

2. Model development

The methodological framework for the financial and real option approach assessment of spelt processing alternatives lies within the inter-relation of the organic spelt processing simulation model KARSIM 1.0 [23]. The first technique presented is one of the common methodological approaches to farm management, while the real option approach is based on the Black-Scholes and binominal models.

2.1. KARSIM 1.0 integrated technologic-economic deterministic simulation model

Simulation modelling can be efficiently applied in both cost estimation and cost benefit analysis [6, 27]. Furthermore, simulation represents one of the fundamental tools for making management decisions [12]. The computer simulation model KARSIM 1.0 was developed for the financial and technological analysis of food processing (organic and conventional).The system as a whole represents a complex calculation system and each sub-model results in a specific enterprise budget. Through a special interface, the system enables simulation of different alternatives at a farm level. Furthermore, based on enterprise budgets, cash flow projections can be conducted together with investment costs for each spelt business alternative, and the net present values for each simulated alternative can be computed. All iterations (calculations for individual alternative) are saved into a database, which is finally used as one of the data sources for real option analysis. The simulation system is built in an Excel spread sheet environment in order to ensure better functionality of a user friendly calculation system. The model structure is presented in Figure 1.

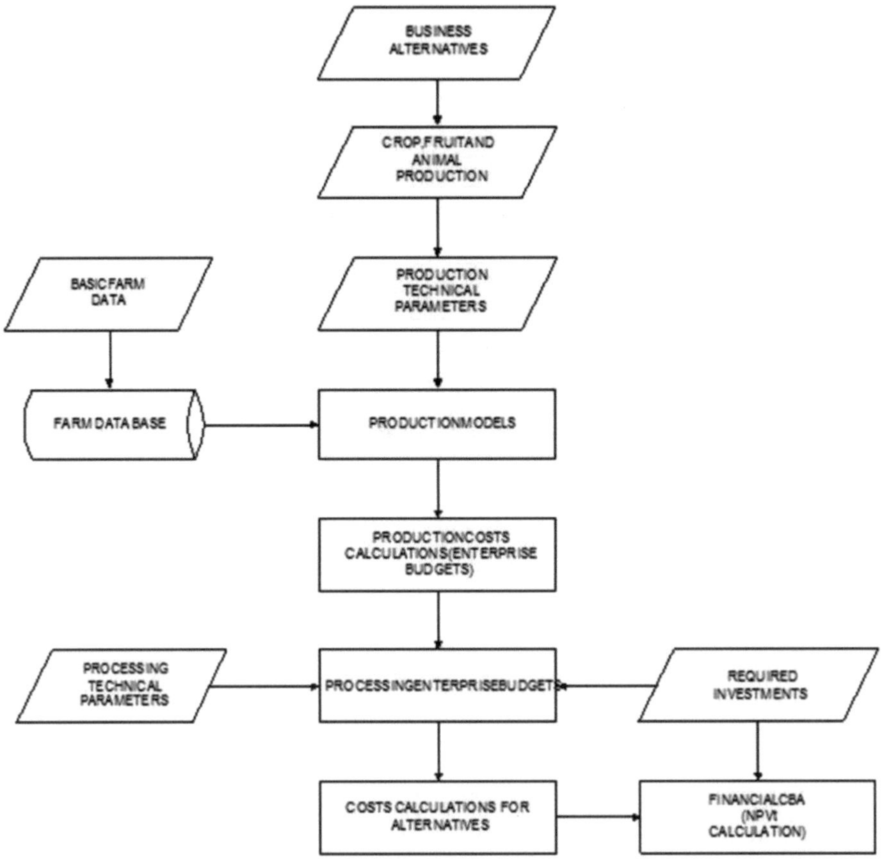

Figure 1. The structure of deterministic simulation model for cost calculations and planning on organic farms KARSIM 1.0.

As presented, the KARSIM 1.0 model is based upon deterministic technologic-economic simulation where the technical relations in the system are expressed with a set of equations or with functional relationships. The amounts of inputs used are calculated as a function of given production intensity, while spelt production costs are calculated as products between the model's estimated inputs usage and their prices. Furthermore, based on enterprise budgets, cash flow projections can be conducted together with the investment costs for each business alternative, and the NPV_t for each simulated alternative can be computed.

2.2. The standard Net Present Value (NPV_t) analysis versus the real options approach

The decision as to which spelt processing method to undertake on an individual farm is rarely made on the basis of NPV_t calculation alone. At this point, we can introduce real option methodology into the planning process where some further KARSIM 1.0 results represent input variables for Black-Scholes and binomial model analysis. The preferred approach to evaluating investments is NPV_tanalysis. For an investment of t periods the formula is:

$$NPV_t = -I + \sum_{i=1}^{n} \frac{TR - TC}{(1+r)^2} \quad (1)$$

Where:

NPV_t - standard Net Present Value (€)

I - investment costs (€)

TR - total revenue (€)

TC - total costs (€)

r - interest rate (%)

t - time - number of years [30].

According to the standard CBA approach, it was presumed that the maximization of the Net Present Value (NPV_t) of the project investment used market prices for expenditures and commodities and describes the financial feasibility. The Net Present Value (NPV_t) parameter is most commonly used in the evaluation of investments in specific investment projects. However, the basic objective of financial analysis is the Net Present Value (NPV). By isolating the cash costs from enterprise budgets, the annual cash flows are estimated, representing a basic input parameter for the computation of NPV_t. In NPV_t equation, the aggregate benefitsTR and the aggregate costs TC are annually summed and discounted to the present with the selected discount rate r.

With isolation of cash costs from enterprise budgets the annual cash flows are estimated, representing a basic input parameter for computation of NPV_t. In equation, where NPV_t is presented, the aggregate benefits SP and the aggregate costs SS are annually summed and discounted to the present with the selected discount rate r. If the sum is positive, investment generatesmore benefits than costs to the project manager (in our case the farmer) and vice versa if the sum is negative. If the NPV_t of the investment after discounting is positive then this investment is better than the alternative earnings. However, in the continuation the concept of options will be introduced how the real options can be appended to the basic NPV_t model.

2.3. Black-Scholes model (BS)

To illustrate the real options methodology, two examples of developed real options model organic spelt processing output are presented, i.e., the Black-Scholes and the binomial models for organic spelt processing business alternatives were developed. Real option describes an option to buy or sell an investment in physical or intangible assets rather than in financial assets. Thus, any corporate investment in plant, equipment, land, patents, brand names, for example, can be the assets on which real options are written. In addition, the investments could be evaluated as real options. Investment (real) opportunities could be treated analogically as financial options. The value of real options is described by the best known Black-Scholes option model (BSOPM)[2]. The link between investments and Black-Scholes inputs are presented in Figure 2.

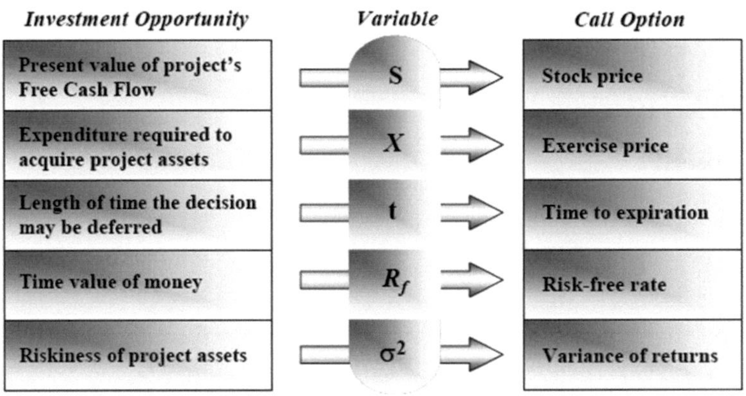

Figure 2. The connections between investments opportunity and Black-Scholes inputs [14].

However, the BS model is one of the most outstanding models in financial economics. The BSOPM based on stochastic calculus is shown below:

$$OV = SN(d_1) - X / e^{-rt}N(d_2) \tag{2}$$

$$d_1 = \left[\ln(S/X) + \left(r_f + ½\, \sigma^2\right) * t \right] / \sigma\sqrt{t} \tag{3}$$

$$d_2 = d_1 - \sigma \sqrt{t} \tag{4}$$

Where:

OV - option value (€),

S - present value of cash flows from optional investment (€),

d_1 - lognormal distribution of $N(d_1)$,

d_2 - lognormal distribution of $N(d_2)$, X - investment expenditure (€),

r_f- annual risk free continuously compounded rate (%),

σ - annualized variance (risk) of the investment's project, t - period until investment (years),

e^{-rt}- the exponential term = 2,71828.

The real options method explicitly accounts for uncertainty in the determination of an optimal decision in light of the stochasticity of an asset's value. The stochastic variable is in calculus expressed in the concept of annual risk free continuously compounded rate and annualized variance (risk) of the investment's project. In the presented case, some of stochastic variables could be defined as risk and uncertainly variables too. Example, the agriculture policy has an important role on organic spelt grain production at this moment.

$$\text{Option value OV} = SN(d_1) - \text{present value of X times } N(d_2) \tag{5}$$

Where$N(d_1)$ and $N(d_2)$ represent the probability distributions. The values of $N(d_1)$ and $N(d_2)$ are obtained from normal probability distribution tables. They give us the probability that S or X will be below d_1 and d_2. In the BS model, they measure the risk associated with the volatility of the value of S.

However, the strategic real options of the investment project are calculated using the Black-Scholes methodology and is calculated as:

$$NPV_{SRO} = NPV_t + OV \tag{6}$$

Where NPV_{SRO}-strategic real option (€).

2.4. The binomial model

The binomial option-pricing model is currently the most widely used real options valuation method. The binomial model (i.e., lattice) describes price movements over time, where the asset value can move to one of two possible prices with associated probabilities [32]. The binomial model is based on a replicating portfolio that combines risk-free borrowing (lending) with the underlying asset to create the same cash flows as the option. Figure 3 represents the binomial process through a decision tree. Since an option represents the right but not the obligation to make an investment, the payoff scheme for the option is asymmetric. The analysis performed in this work makes use of the multiplicative binomial model of Cox and Rubinstein [5], the standard tool for option pricing in discrete time.

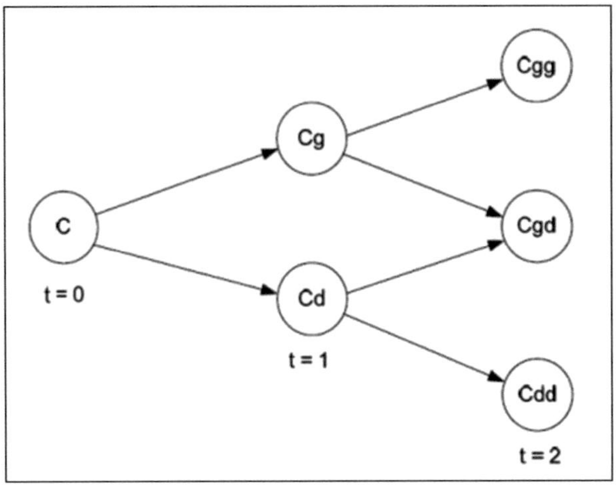

Figure 3. Binominal lattice structure (C= NPV_t with probability d_1 = Cg and d_2 = Cd; Cgg = Cg * d_1, Cgd = Cd * d_1 and Cdd = Cd * d_2).

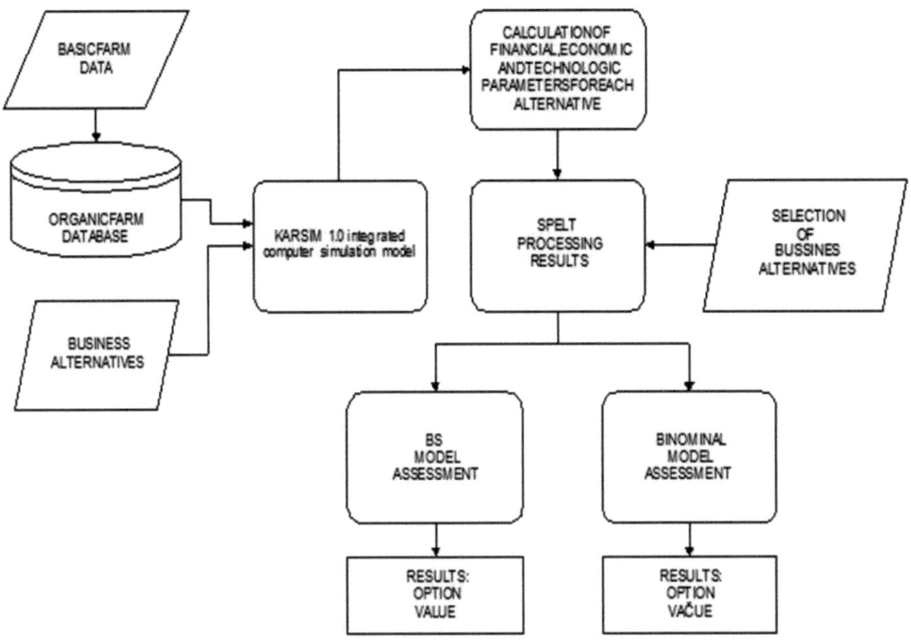

Figure 4. Decision Support Structure for organic spelt processing and option value calculation.

According to Figure 3, a node of value C= NPV_t can lead to two nodes with their values being given by C= NPV_t with probability 1+d = d_1= Cg and 1-d = d_2 = Cd, respectively. Thus, the lattice provides a representation of all possible demand values throughout the whole project life [7]. The investment project option value (OV) could be calculated using the backward induction process [28, 33].

In the next part, for easier understanding of assessments operation and models functionality, the cumulative structure of integrated decision support system for organic spelt processing alternatives and its option values calculation is in details presented in Figure 4.

However, the goal of integrated model development is to provide answers which business alternative is the best solution for the given sample organic farm.

3. Case study

In the chapter the application of the presented methodology in the context of organic spelt processing investments alternatives is presented.An organic part time-farm with 5,1 ha of arable land in north eastern Slovenia was considered in order to compare spelt processing investment projects using the real option models methodology. The presented farm regularly includes besides other grains spelt wheat (*TriticumspeltaL.*) in its crop rotation. The basic characteristic of spelt wheat is its high resistance to diseases, and low input of nitrogen. On the other perspective, spelt wheat can be directly processed into different kinds of food products on the farm itself, and represents additional business and market opportunities for organic farmers. However, the annual area of spelt wheat is, according to crop rotation rules, limited to 1 ha with an average yield of 2500 kg unhusked spelt grain (the average yield/ha on Slovene organic farms). The service of husking and milling the grain is outsourced by the farmer and is calculated as variable cost. Spelt is used for animal fodder, but the alternative option considered in this model is to produce and sell spelt grain and spelt flour to individual customers for human nutrition.

4. Results and discussion

The identified business alternatives are evaluated using a specially developed simulation models in Excel spreadsheet environment. Basic production data and calculated economical parameters for individual business alternatives in spelt processing are presented in Table 1.

Based on discounted cash flow methodology, the traditional net present value (NPV_t) criterion is used extensively in assessing an investment opportunity for three analysed spelt products (table 2).The results are calculated under the assumption of successful product selling at the expected prices. The estimated production levels were calculated on the basis of the annual spelt production area. As shown in table 2, CBA analysis shows positive net present values for both processed spelt for human nutrition (spelt grain and spelt flour). The highest NPV_t was observed for husked spelt grain (NPV_t = 9.224,84 €). The relatively high estimated NPV_t for spelt grain can be explained by high prices, achieved in the market. The negative

NPV_t was calculated for spelt grain for animal nutrition and is expected (the price on the market is compared to husked spelt grain for human nutrition lower, but on the other hand the basic production costs are the same as by processed spelt grain). The investment return period (Pd) is for husked spelt grain and spelt flour 2 years. However, the corresponding NPV_t by Pd is for husked spelt grain (human nutrition) higher compared to spelt flour (NPV_t= 2.482,12 € and NPV_t= 1.066,96 €).

Business alternative	Products quantity** (kg)	Total costs (€)	Total revenue (€)	Coefficient of economics
Husked spelt* (animal fodder)	1.688,00	478,00	591,15	1,24
Husked spelt grain (human nutrition)	1.688,00	1.495,30	4.389,25	2,94
Spelt flour	1.350,00	1.675,15	3.795,05	2,27

*on Slovene organic farms is spelt usually used in animal feed rations as husked spelt
**products quantity based on annual spelt average yield/ha on Slovene organic farms

Table 1. The simulation model results for the planned spelt processing projects on a sample farm.

Product	Investment costs (€)	Annual cash flow (€)	NPV_t (€)	Investment return period=Pd (years)	NPV_t by Pd (€)
Spelt grain (animal nutrition)	580,00	113,19	-128,08	/	/
Spelt grain (human nutrition)	2.960,00	3.051,77	9.224,84	2	2.482,12
Spelt flour	2.960,00	2.259,19	6.056,31	2	1.066,96

Table 2. Financial CBA analysis of the planned spelt processing projects on a sample farm (after 5 years, discount rate = 8%).

However, as expected, the investment into spelt grain for animal fodder is financial unfeasible (NPV_t = -128,97€) and investment return period is not possible to assessed. From financial aspect this project should be rejected. Further, the results of traditional Net Present Value for spelt grain production (animal fodder) presents the base for calculation of strategic real option of spelt grain (for human nutrition) and spelt flour. The risk-free rate and variance of the investment's project were defined deterministic. To illustrate the real options methodology, we present two examples of our real options model output. In the first part of tables 3 and 4 the parameters used in the real options model calculation for the spelt grain and spelt flour production are demonstrated. In the second part of the table 3 and 4 there are calculated simulation models results for real options calculation.

Parameters description	Value
Present Value of cash flows from optional investment (€)	3.051,77
Investment expenditure (€)	2.960,00
Exponential function	2,71828
Risk-free rate (%)	8,00
Period until investment (years)	5
Variance (Risk) of the investment's project (%)	50
d1	0,9440974
d2	-0,173936588
Lognormal distribution of d1	0,827440061
Lognormal distribution of d2	0,430957649
Option value of spelt grain (human nutrition)(€)	1.670,07
Strategic real option of spelt grain for animal nutrition (processing of spelt grain for human nutrition) (€)	1.541,99

Table 3. Descriptions and values of parameters for the real options model for spelt grain (human nutrition).

As seen in table 3, option value for husked spelt grain, calculated by Black-Scholes methodology, is 1.670,07 €. Further, the strategic real option of spelt grain (animal nutrition) is a positive value too. The results of the application of BS methodology by analysed farm business alternative showed the interest in investment project (strategic real option = 1.541,99 €) and is suggested to accept the project.

Parameters description	Value
Present Value of cash flows from optional investment (€)	2.258,19
Investment expenditure (€)	2.960,00
Exponential function	2,71828
Risk-free rate (%)	8
Period until investment (years)	5
Variance (Risk) of the investment's project (%)	50
d1	0,674733898
d2	-0,443300091
Lognormal distribution of d1	0,750077578
Lognormal distribution of d2	0,328774345
Option value of spelt flour (human nutrition)(€)	1.041,48
Strategic real option of spelt grain for animal nutrition (processing in spelt flour)(€)	913,40

Table 4. Descriptions and values of parameters for the real options model for spelt flour.

The results of analysed farm business alternative (spelt flour, Table 4) indicate that the calculated option value is 1.041,48 €. According to the option value calculation, the strategic real option of spelt grain for animal nutrition and further processing into spelt flour is a bit lower value as by processing into spelt grain for human nutrition, but in analysed case again the positive value (SRO = 913,40€). Under the model assumptions,the spelt flour production option is suitable and financial interesting for the farmer.

On the basis of calculated data with BS methodology it can be concluded, that under presumed input parameters both business alternative are for the farmer suitable option.

Further, investment project option values are calculated using the binomial lattice too. However, the results of real options approach show more favourable picture from farmers' perspective by binominal model. The results showed that financially the most interesting and suitable investment is spelt grain for human nutrition where the option value results in a value of 2.678,81 € followed by spelt flour production (1.577,37€). All binomial model results are calculated under the assumption presented in Table 5.

Parameter	Spelt grain (human nutrition)	Spelt flour
OV (€)	2.678,81	1.577,37

Table 5. Option value assessments for spelt processing using binominal model.

upfactord$_1$ = 1,648720716

down factord$_2$ = 0,606530864

p = 0,457456139

1-p = 0,542543861

The detailed presentation of the binomial lattice calculations is in Table 6 to Table 9.

Time (years)	*0*	*1*	*2*	*3*	*4*	*5*
OV (€)	3.051,77	5.031,52	8.296,57	1.3677,08	22.549,68	37.178,14
		1.850,99	3.051,77	5.031,52	8.295,57	13.677,09
			1.122,68	1.850,99	3.051,77	5.031,52
				680,94	1.122,68	1.850,99
					413,01	680,94
						250,50

Table 6. Asset valuation lattice for spelt grain for human nutrition using binominal model (for first 5 years of production).

As seen previously in all cases, is the most suitable alternative production spelt grain for human consumption. It should be mentioned that there are between both model results differences in the individual alternative assessments. The presented results showed that binominal models further confirm the preliminary CBA results (Table 2).

Time (years)	*0*	*1*	*2*	*3*	*4*	*5*
OV (€)	2.678,81	5.208,81	8.432,14	13.639,89	19.589,68	34.218,14
		956,82	1.827,69	3.290,62	5.335,57	10.717,09
			155,99	369,40	874,77	2.071,52
				0,00	0,00	0,00
					0,00	0,00
						0,00

Table 7. Option value assessments for spelt grainwith binominal model (for first 5 years of production).

Time (years)	*0*	*1*	*2*	*3*	*4*	*5*
OV (€)	2.258,19	3.723,12	6.138,39	10.120,50	16.685,88	27.510,37
		1.369,66	2.258,19	3.723,13	6.138,40	10.120,51
			830,74	1.369,66	2.258,19	3.723,13
				503,61	830,74	1.369,66
					305,61	503,87
						185,36

Table 8. Asset valuation lattice for spelt flour for human nutrition using binominal model (for first 5 years of production).

Time (years)	*0*	*1*	*2*	*3*	*4*	*5*
OV (€)	1.577,37	3.208,96	5.553,91	9.382,44	13.725,88	24.550,37
		443,81	889,58	1.724,39	3.178,40	7.160,51
			57,47	136,08	322,26	763,13
				0,00	0,00	0,00
					0,00	0,00
						0,00

Table 9. Option value assessments for spelt flour with binominal model (for first 5 years of production).

However, the model results showed that both project results with positive values. But it should be mentioned that does not mean that the project may be accepted and invested immediately. It should be taken into account the flexibility and possible options. The positive option values means that the farmer should hold the option of analyzed project investment and do not abandon the project simply.

5. Conclusion

The application of discount cash flow approach in agriculture is not always the appropriate way to decide if an investment project is feasible or not. In the paper, an attempt was made to employ a real options approach to evaluate the spelt processing business alternatives on a farm. The general implication from this empirical analysis is that uncertainty and risk attitudes play an important role in farmers' decision to adopt a new business. Empirical results reveal that the production of spelt grain for animal fodder versus spelt grain (for human nutrition) and spelt flour is not advisable for the analysed farm. The model results are useful in practice and helpful in setting up hedges in the correct proportions to minimize risk. However, real option approach offers a new point of view to investment evaluation of agri-food project. The option methodology takes into account uncertain parameters, forecasting and the most important, the value of opportunity. We can conclude, that real options are comprehensive and integrated solution to apply options theory to value real investments project to improve the decision making process.

Author details

Karmen Pažek* and Črtomir Rozman *

*Address all correspondence to: karmen.pazek@uni-mb.si

Chair of Agricultural Economics and Rural Development/University of Maribor/Faculty of Agriculture and Life Sciences/Pivola, Slovenia

References

[1] Amram, M., & Kulatilaka, N. (1999). *Real Options: Managing Strategic Investment in an Uncertain World*, Boston, Massachusetts, Harvard Business School Press.

[2] Black, F., & Scholes, M. (1973). The Pricing of Options and Corporate Liabilities. *Journal of Political Economy*, 81(5-6), 637.

[3] Brennan, M., & Schwartz, E. (1985). Evaluating natural resource investments. *Business*, 58135-157.

[4] Collins, R., & Hanf, C. H. (1998). Evaluation of farm investments: Biases in Net Present Value estimates from using quasi-deterministic models in an uncertain world. *Agricultural Finance Review*, 58-81.

[5] Cox, J. C. , & Rubinstein, M. (1990). Option Pricing: A Simplified Approach. *Financial Econ.*, 1979, 7229-263, reprinted in The Handbook of Financial Engineering, Harper Business Publishers.

[6] Csaki, C. (1985). *Simulation and System Analysis in Agriculture*, Amsterdam, Elsevier.

[7] Dalila-Fontes, B. M. M. (2008). Fixed versus flexible production systems: A real options analysis. *European Journal of Operational Research*, 188169-184.

[8] Dixit, A., & Pindyck, R. (1994). *Investment Under Uncertainty*, Princeton, NJ, Princeton University Press.

[9] Ekboir, J. M. (1997). Technical change and irreversible investment under risk. *Agricultural Economics*, 16(1), 54-65.

[10] Hadelan, L., Njavro, M., & Par, V. (2008). Option Models in Investment Appraisal. 43rd Croatian & 3rd International Symposium on Agriculture. *Book of Abstracts*, 47-48.

[11] Khanna, M., Isik, M., & Winter-Nelson, A. (2000). Investment in site-specific crop management under uncertainty: implications for nitrogen pollution control and environmental policy. *Agriculture Economics*, 249-21.

[12] Kljajić, M., Bernik, I., & Škraba, A. (2000). Simulation approach to decision assessment in enterprises. *Simulation*, 75(4), 199-210.

[13] Kuminoff, N., & Wossink, A. (2010). Why isn't more US farmland Organic? *Journal of Agricultural Economics*, 61(2), 240-258.

[14] Leuhrman, T. (1998). Investment Opportunities as Real Options. *Harvard Business Review*.

[15] Morgan, D. G., Abdallah, S. B., & Lasserre, P. (2007). A Real Options Approach to Forest-Management Decision Making to Protect Caribou under the Threat of Extinction. *Ecology and Society*.

[16] Musshoff, O. (2012). Growing short rotation coppice on agricultural land in Germany: A Real Options Approach. *Biomass and Bioenergy*, 41-73.

[17] Musshoff, N. H. (2008). Adoption of organic farming in Germany and Austria: An integrative dynamic investment perspective. *Agricultural Economics*, 39-135.

[18] Musshoff, O., & Odening, M. (2005, June 22-25). Adoption of Organic Farming. Real Options, Theory Meets Practice. Paris- France. *9th Annual International Conference*.

[19] Nadolnyak, D., Miranda, M. J., & Sheldon, I. (2011). *International Journal of Industrial Organization*, 29-455.

[20] Nishihara, M., & Fukushima, M. (2008). Evaluation of firm's loss due to incomplete information in real investment decision. *European Journal of Operational Research*, 188569-585.

[21] Pandza, K., Horsburgh, S., Gorton, K., & Polajnar, A. (2003). A real options approach to managing resources and capabilities Inter J. *Operations & Production Management*, 23(9), 1010-1032.

[22] Pažek, K., & Rozman, Č. (2011). Business opportunity assessment in Slovene organic spelt processing: application of real options model. *Renewable agriculture and food systems*, 26(3), 179-184.

[23] Pažek, K. (2006). Integrated computer simulation model KARSIM 1.0. *Internal database*, University of Maribor, Faculty of Agriculture and Life Sciences, Slovenia.

[24] Pažek, K., Rozman, Č., Borec, A., Turk, J., Majkovič, D., Bavec, M., & Bavec, F. (2006). The use of multi criteria models for decision support on organic farms. *Biological Agriculture and Horticulture*, 24(1), 73-89.

[25] Price, T. J., & Wetzstein, M. E. (1999). Irreversible investment decisions in perennial crops with yield and price uncertainty. *Journal of Agricultural and Resource Economic*, 24-173.

[26] Purvis, A., Boggess, W. G., Moss, C. B., & Holt, J. (1996). Technology adoption decisions under irreversibility and uncertainty: An Ex Ante approach. *American Journal of Agricultural Economics*, 541-551.

[27] Rozman, Č., Tojnko, S., Turk, J., Par, V., & Pavlovič, M. (2002). Die Anwendungeines Computersimulationsmodellszur Optimierung der Erweiterungeiner Apfelplantageunter den Bedingungen der Republik Slowenien. *Berichteüber Landwirtscahft*, 80(4), 632-642.

[28] Rozman, Č., Pažek, K., Bavec, M., Bavec, F., Turk, J., & Majkovič, D. (2006). The Multi-criteria analysis of spelt food processing alternatives on small organic farms. *Journal of Sustainable Agriculture*, 28159-179.

[29] Tegene, A., Wiebe, K., & Kuhn, B. (1999). Irreversible investment under uncertainty: Conservation easements and the option to develop agricultural land. *Journal of Agricultural Economics*, 50(2), 203-219.

[30] Turk, J., & Rozman, Č. (2002). A feasibility study of fruit brandy production. *Agricultura*, 1(1), 28-33.

[31] Tzouramani, I., & Mattas, K. (2009). Evaluating Economic Incentives for Greek Organic Agriculture: A Real Options Approach. Ed. Rezitis, A. E-book series, Research Topics in Agricultural and Applied Economics. *Benthan Science Publishers*, 1-23.

[32] Wang, Z., & Tang, X. (2010). Research of Investment Evaluation of Agricultural Venture Capital Project on real Options Approach. *Agriculture and Agricultural science Procedia*, 1-449.

[33] Winter-Nelson, A., & Amegbeto, K. (1998). Option values to conservation and agricultural price policy: Application to terrace construction in Kenya. *American Journal of Agricultural Economics*, 80409-418.

Section 2

Organic Food Quality and Sustainability

Chapter 4

The Quality of Organically Produced Food

Ewa Rembiałkowska, Aneta Załęcka,
Maciej Badowski and Angelika Ploeger

Additional information is available at the end of the chapter

http://dx.doi.org/10.5772/54525

1. Introduction

Organic farming began to develop in the modern world as a response to intensified farming and industrial agriculture, using synthetic fertilizers, chemical pesticides, introduction of monocultures into large areas, the separation the animal husbandry from plant production and using heavy machinery. All of this leads both to environmental degradation, and on the other hand, the overproduction of food. At the same time the food quality decreases continuously with regard to nutritional value, which is also the effect of strongly developed food technology.

Regulations specifying the conditions of organic crop and animal production are very strict, which results in high quality of agricultural products. The same applies to the processing scheme, however the techniques are not regulated so far (only few ones, such as radiation and genetic modifications, are banned in organic food processing). While conventional processing is based on several hundred different types of food additives (colorings, stabilizers, enhancers, etc.), the organic food processing allows only few dozen of additives, which usually are natural substances. This is a particularly difficult situation for organic farmers, who are obliged to maintain the quality of their products without using chemicals. However, the consumers' health is essential.

2. Food quality

The quality of food products is a subject of many debates, which result in different definitions of this term. The definition of food quality is constantly changing. Initially it was represented by the quantitative/measurable parameters. Nowadays more and more popular is the holistic approach to the problem of quality. Vogtmann (1991) adopted a food quality evaluation approach including analytical and holistic criteria. According to this approach, the organic food quality assessment should be focused on all aspects and from all possible points of view, i.e. holistic model. Kahl et al., (2010a) analyzed the current status of organic food quality in relation to potential quality claims. They concluded, that a model is missed, which can be applied in scientific research as well as in practice. Furthermore they identified a gap between consumer expectations on the quality of the food and what can be guaranteed by regulation so far. Recently Kahl et al., (2012) published a model for organic food quality, taking into account a conceptual background which consists of the different (historical) sources as IFOAM standards, EC-Regulations and consumer understanding. A central part of this model is the evaluation, which should take part on different levels. As am essential part, organic food quality consists of product and process related aspects, which can be described by criteria and measured by parameters. This holistic or systemic view brings all different criteria together: technological value, nutritional value, sensory value as well as biological value and ethical indicators.

The technological value refers to the distinctive features of food products in light of the requirements of different interest groups. For individual participants of the food production chain (producers, processors, distributors and consumers) different features may be the most important distinguishing parameters, depending on the specific purpose for which the food product is intended.

The sensory quality is represented by a set of features assessed by humans by the use of standarized tests, based on human senses: taste, smell, touch, vision and hearing. Among these criteria, the appearance plays an important role in the assessment of raw materials and finished products, along with other organoleptic characteristics such as taste, smell or texture. Sensory quality is of great importance because it affects the process of making a choice when buying food. Sensory evaluation of food products is based on two main methods. The first one is to assess the desirability, acceptance and consumer preferences assessed in so-called 'consumer tests'. The second method is to evaluate the product based on defined criteria and by a specially trained person (so-called 'sensory panel'). The results are analyzed statistically.

The nutritional value can be considered as the minimum content of food contaminants (pesticide residues, nitrates, heavy metals, etc.) at the optimum content of valuable ingredients (vitamins, mineral elements, protein, etc.)

Interestingly the quality of organic food is mainly measured by standard single compound detection through analytical methods. In order to follow the holistic view on agriculture, also the evaluation of the food should be more holistic than reductionistic. Kahl et al., (2010 b) discussed several approaches and methods for this purpose. The biocrystallization method seems to be most encouraging in this direction (Kahl et al., 2009, Szulc et al., 2010, Busscher et al., 2010a,b).

Another question, related to organic food quality is, how authentic the food is. Authenticity can be understood in two ways. First one is represented by the sense of product traceability, when it is possible to verify whether the characteristics of the product actually correspond to characteristics that are attributed to him. For instance, research conducted to determine whether the products offered on the market as organic really come from organic production (Kahl et al., 2010b). Therefore, it is needed to find methods that would enable tracing of all "biography of the product" in a fast and simple way. It would be an efficient tool for controlling the products offered on the market. Here an European project, bringing several approaches together is currently working on this topic (www.http://www.coreorganic2.org/Upload/CoreOrganic2/Document/Leaflet_AuthenticFood_2012.pdf) and the second approach authenticity can be understood as a counterweight to the growing trend of food globalization. More and more people look for food from safe sources, produced locally by the well-known manufacturers. Nowadays, food is transported from long distances, from the place of production by the place of processing up to the point of sale. As a result, consumers look for products less intensively processed, derived from known safe sources such as buying locally and directly from the farmer. The average food transport route from the place of production to the place of consumption in America is approximately 2,000 km (Wilkins and Gussow, 1997). There are scientific studies showing that it is possible to satisfy the nutritional needs of consumers with the State of New York based mainly on food produced locally. On the other hand, local agriculture in this state disappeared almost completely, although most consumers of the State of New York evaluated the local varieties of vegetables and fruits better (Wilkins and Gussow, 1997). The active opposition against food globalization is represented by the movement called "slow food" - to support food production which is an alternative to "fast food".

The biological value defines the impact of food on human health. This criterion is based on the holistic approach to the food quality and on the belief that the knowledge of the chemical composition of foods is not sufficient to determine the relationship between the consumed food and the human health. At the same time health is understood not only as the absence of disease, but also as the well-being, fertility and vitality. So far, several scientific studies have been conducted with regard to this issue, but only on laboratory animals (mice, rats and rabbits). Due to many obstacles of a formal, logistic and economic nature, very few studies assessing the direct impact of organic food on human health have been carried out.

The ethical value of food quality comprise three aspects: the aspect of environmental impact, the socio-economic aspect and the farm animal welfare.

One of the main factors determining the quality of products is the quality of the environment. We can expect the best crop quality only where the air, soil, ground-and surface water meet the required quality standards. Legal regulations on organic farming does not provide specific guidance on the definition of the quality of the agricultural environment where organic production can take place. However, the guidelines elaborated by various associations of organic farming may specify requirements in this field. Organic farmers are required to maintain the environment in good condition and should try to support the cycle approach. The organic production methods are focused on the protection of all environmental components against the pressure of the agricultural aspects. Environmental impact of organic and conventional farming was researched by Tyburski and Żakowska-Biemans (2007). The authors point out that organic farming consumes less energy, which is of great importance. Nowadays, when the world is focused on energy crisis, organic agriculture achieves lower energy consumption rates because it does not apply fertilizers and pesticides, whose production requires high energy inputs. In addition, high energy lead to large emissions of greenhouse gases and the conventional farming is a very large emission source of them. Therefore, organic plant production significantly contributes to reducing greenhouse gas emissions. Furthermore, conventional agriculture leads to eutrophication and pollution of water resources, i.a. by the use of pesticides (Tyburski and Żakowska-Biemans, 2007). The biological diversity resulting from the spatial complexity of organic agricultural landscape supports three important functions: an ecological function, which is to maintain biological diversity and homeostasis; the production function, based on prevention, rather than fighting diseases and pests; and the function of the health and welfare, which results from the fact that humans are an integral part of the environment and can exist only through the harmonious coexistence with nature. Contact with nature is essential for mental health, and mental health is the foundation of physical health.

The choice of agricultural products, which are produced, processed and sold under conditions of equality and social justice is becoming increasingly popular among EU consumers. So-called "fair trade" principles implemented within developing countries are very important. By boycotting companies that do not follow the socioeconomic rules, the consumers may have a positive impact on reducing social inequalities, which are common in the production, processing and sale of agricultural products within tropical countries. Consumers have the choice because of the wide access to information about companies in the food trade market.

Furthermore, environmentally aware consumers are now more and more convinced that the methods of animal husbandry are important even during making decisions about purchasing food products. The reason is the suffering of animals, which is a result of very inappropriate conditions of animal husbandry (crowding, aggression, disease).

3. Plant products

3.1. Harmful substances

Pesticides are a group of synthetic compounds which do not occur in nature, and are introduced into environment as a deliberate human decision. Use of pesticides can increase the profitability of crops, protecting them against pests and diseases. However, the applied chemicals do not affect only the target organisms. Their residues accumulate in plants and move along the food chain, including the human body. Depending on the dose consumed by a man with the contaminated food, the consequences include various health effects. In order to reduce the adverse impact of pesticides on human health, the Maximum Residue Limit (MRL) of pesticide, which may be present in food, has been established. MRL is usually established by testing of pesticides on rats. It is believed that the consumption of pesticides below the MRLs does not impose a health risk. However, pesticides even in low concentrations are known or suspected to be the cause of many diseases and health problems including birth defects and cancer (BMA, 1992; Howard, 2005). The main problem is that the MRLs for pesticides are usually determined by testing of individual active substances (each one) on rats for a relatively short period of time. Almost nothing is known about the effects of consuming a total of potentially hundreds of different pesticides during the whole lifetime and associated actions resulting from synergistic mixtures of pesticides. This reaction is named in literature as a 'cocktail effect'. According to Howard (2005), the most recommended way to protect ourselves is to avoid consuming all of pesticides, especially in case of pregnant women, nursing mothers and young children up to 3 years. In 1994-1999 Baker et al., (2002) analyzed in the USA the fruit and vegetables from the three types of production (organic, integrated and conventional) for pesticide residues content. According to the results, the percentage of organic crops with a known presence of pesticide residues was approximately three times lower compared to conventional crops, and about two times lower compared to the raw materials from integrated agriculture (see Figure 1). Most samples with pesticide residues were found in conventional celery, spinach, pears and apples.

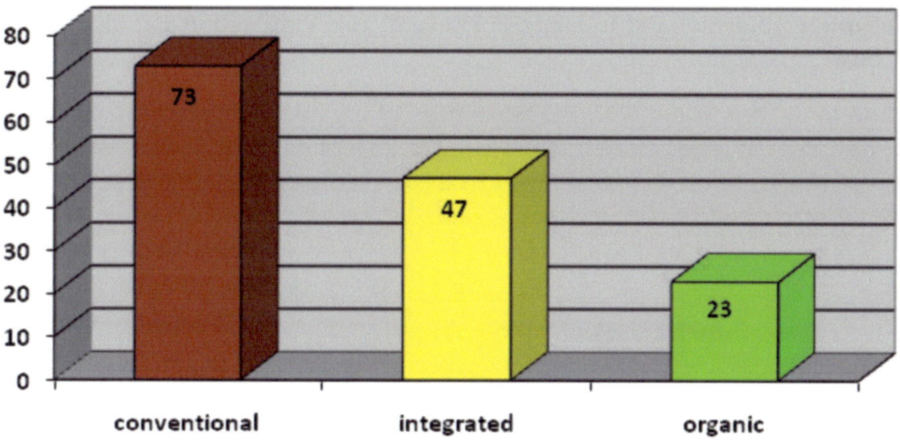

Figure 1. The comparison of contamination of agricultural crops with pesticide residues in the USA (in %) (Baker et al., 2002)

According to Lairon (2010), who reviewed the reports of French Agency of Food Safety and recent studies, from 94 to 100 per cent of organic foodstuffs contain no pesticide residues. In 1995-2001 similar survey was conducted in Belgium. The results revealed, that the percentage of organic crops contaminated with pesticides was 12%, whereas in the case of conventional crops this percentage reached 49% (AFSCA-FAVV, 2001). Research carried out in Poland gave a surprising result, as the highest percentages of crops containing pesticide residues were found in integrated agriculture, i.e. 47% (2005) and 48% (2006). Conventional agriculture presented the intermediate state between the other two management systems - 28% of raw materials in 2005 and 21% in 2006 contained pesticide residues. Crops derived from organic production were contaminated at a level of 5% (2005) and 7% (2006), which were the lowest among all three systems. The detected residues of pesticides in organic fruits and vegetables result from its unauthorized use (Gnusowski and Nowacka, 2007), which indicates the imperfect control system of organic farms conducted by certification bodies. Such situations occur not only in Poland but in all countries worldwide. It should be noted that those cases are rare and in general organic raw materials present much lower pesticide residue level compared to conventional ones. Therefore, it is expected that a diet based on organic products should result in lower levels of pesticides in breast milk and human tissues. A few studies support this hypothesis. It was found in France that pesticide residues in human breast milk decreased significantly with increasing share of organic food (from 25% to 80%) in the daily diet of lactating women (Aubert, 1987). Similar results were obtained by comparing the content of organophosphorus pesticide residues in blood and urine of children fed organically vs. conventionally (Curl et al., 2003). Body fluids of children on conventional diet contained six times more pesticide residues than children on organic diet. These results indicate that consumption of organic products can significantly reduce the risk of excess pesticide intake with food and thus improve public health.

Each year the European Food Safety Authority (EFSA) publishes a report on monitoring of pesticide contamination in the market food in 27 European Union member states and two EFTA countries (Norway and Iceland). For several years, the report has also included the studies on organic food.

According to the report for 2007, the percentage of organic food products containing residues of pesticides at levels exceeding the MRL value was much lower than for conventional products. A similar result was obtained in 2008 (see Figure 2).

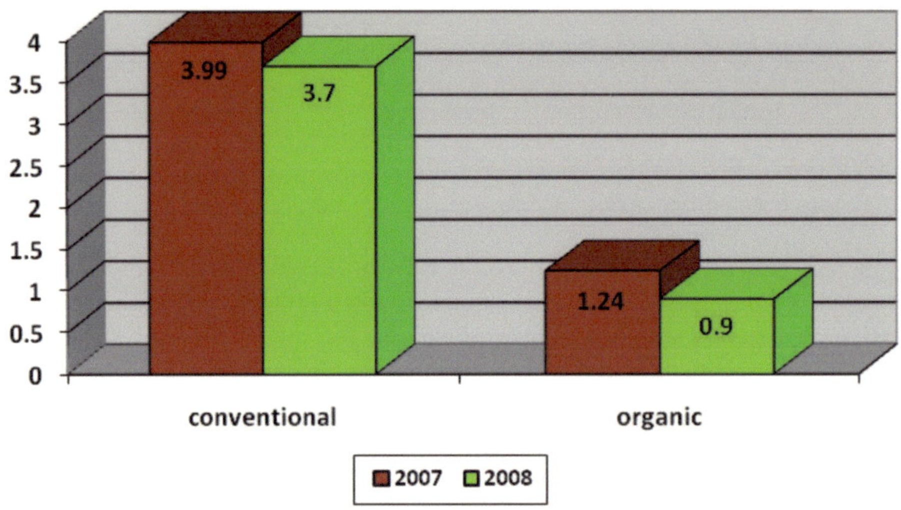

Figure 2. Samples with pesticide residues above the MRL in European food (%) (EFSA, 2009; 2010)

A number of studies clearly indicate a higher content of nitrates and nitrites in conventionally produced crops compared to organic ones. According to Lairon (2010) organic vegetables contain approximately 50% lower levels of nitrites when compared to conventional ones. This is the result of the treatment with synthetic, readily soluble nitrogen fertilizers, that is absorbed in large quantities through the root system and leads to accumulation of nitrates in the leaves and other plant organs. The organic system allows using organic fertilizers, which also contain nitrogen, but in organically bound form. When they reach the soil, followed by further decomposition of the fertilizer by soil microorganisms and by edaphon, the complex organic-mineral compound (humus) is formed. The plants get nitrogen from the humus only when they need it, so there is little possibility of excessive accumulation of nitrate in plant organs (Vogtmann, 1985). This is important for human health because the nitrates are converted into nitrites, which can cause a dangerous condition known as methemoglobinemia in case of infants, young children and older people (Mirvish, 1993). Furthermore, nitrite can react with amines to form carcinogenic and mutagenic nitrosamines, causing gastrointestinal cancers and leukemia (Szponar and Kierzkowska, 1990). This process is dangerous not only for children but also for adults of any age. Many authors compared the nitrate content in organic vs. conventional crops in the following species: white cabbage (Wawrzyniak et al., 2004; Rutkowska, 1999; Rembiałkowska, 2000), red cabbage (Rutkowska, 1999), potatoes (Hajslova et al., 2005; Rembiałkowska, 2000; Rembiałkowska, 1998), lettuce (Guadagnin et al., 2005), beetroot (Leszczyńska, 1996; Rembiałkowska, 2000), parsley (Rutkowska, 1999), carrot (Rembiałkowska, 1998; Rutkowska, 1999; Rembiałkowska, 2000), celery (Wawrzyniak et al., 2004), Pac Choy Chinese cabbage (Wawrzyniak et al., 2004). After averaging the results of the above studies and application of a formula by Worthington (2001): (CONV-ORG) / ORG x 100%, conventional crops contain an average of 148.39% more nitrate than organic crops. The highest levels of nitrate were found in red beetroots, because they exhibit the tendency of nitrate accumulation in roots. Therefore, despite their high nutritional value we should pay particular attention to the production system, as the best choice is the organic agriculture. The data presented above provide a basis to conclude that organic system helps to reduce the intake of nitrates and nitrites by the human body.

Heavy metals such as cadmium, lead, arsenic, mercury and zinc are introduced into the food chain from various sources: industry, transport, municipal waste and agriculture. For example, mineral phosphate fertilizers used in conventional agriculture can introduce cadmium into plant crops, as well as the metal industry and transportation cause cadmium contamination of soil and crops. Therefore, there are no clear differences in the heavy metal content between organic and conventional raw materials. Some of the studies confirm the higher levels of heavy metals in conventional crops, whereas other authors show the opposite results (Rembiałkowska, 2000). Problem to be solved is whether organic farming (composting, increasing of soil organic matter, increasing soil pH, etc.) can reduce the intake of heavy metals by crops.

Mycotoxins are toxic compounds produced by fungi of the groups of *Aspergillus*, *Penicillium* and *Fusarium*, which are found in food products (Kouba, 2003). Production of mycotoxins depends primarily on temperature, humidity and other environmental conditions. The effect of mycotoxins consumption on human health is negative, as they perform carcinogenic properties and affect negatively the immune system. More and more studies are currently carried out in order to compare the content of mycotoxins in food products, as the consumers are becoming more aware of aspects concerning food safety. The content of mycotoxins in organic products is discussed all over the world, as the use of fungicides in organic farming is prohibited. The most important question is whether the system of agricultural production has an impact on the development of mycotoxins. Studies comparing the mycotoxins content in organic vs. conventional products show comparable amounts in both types of products, sometimes indicating lower content of mycotoxins in organic products. Spadaro et al., (2006) and Versari et al., (2007) confirmed lower amounts of mycotoxins in organic products compared to conventional ones. Even if the level of mycotoxins in organic products is higher, the differences are small and do not exceed acceptable levels (Gottschalk et al., 2007; Jestoi, 2004; Pussemier, 2004; Maeder et al., 2007). According to Lairon (2010), organic cereals contain similar levels of mycotoxins as conventional cereals. An important case is wheat, which is a commonly consumed grain in European countries (mostly in the form of bread and pasta), and may be contaminated with mycotoxins. For this reason, much research is done to ensure the food security of winter wheat. The studies revealed that the level of damage caused by *Fusarium* and the concentration of mycotoxins were lower in case of organic crops. Environmental factors have comparable impact on the content of mycotoxins as the use of varieties with high resistance (Wieczyńska, 2010).

3.2. Bioactive substances

The nutritional value of food depends primarily on the appropriate content of compounds necessary for the proper functioning of the human body. The content of phytochemicals in plant foods is a major concern in the current food science. Secondary plant metabolites play a critical role in human health and may have a very high nutritional value (Lundegårdh and Mårtensson, 2003). Phenolic compounds are of particular interest because of their potential antioxidant activity and other healthy properties, including properties that may prevent cancer (Brandt and Mølgaard, 2001). Therefore the content of the secondary metabolites from the group of phenolic compounds in plant foods is of great interest, as more and more scientific studies are focused on comparing their content in organic and conventional products.

Secondary plant metabolites are substances naturally synthesized by the plant, but usually do not take direct part in the creation of its cells. They are usually produced as a reaction to exposure of the plant on the external stimuli, performing the functions of physiological changes regulators in case of pests attack or other stress factors (Brandt and Mølgaard, 2001). These substances include antioxidants, which protect the organism against the effects of many external factors and reduce the risk of civilization diseases (Di Renzo et al., 2007).

Plant secondary metabolites can be basically divided into compounds that do not contain nitrogen phenolic compounds, such as phenolic acids, flavonoids (six classes of them: flavones, flavonols, flavanones, flavanols, isoflavones, anticyanides) and terpenoids (e.g.

tetraterpenes, carotenes, xanthophylls) and nitrogen-containing compounds (alkaloids, amines, non-protein amino acids, glycosides, glucosinolates).

Mostly discussed are flavonoids, which constitute a large group of several thousand different compounds and play an important role in healthcare, performing many functions in the human body (Bidlack, 1998). Flavonoids present strong antioxidant activity, they chelate metals, affect the immune system e.g. by inhibiting tumor growth, prevent arteriosclerosis, strengthens blood vessel walls, reduce blood clot formation and thus reduce the risk of stroke, have a protective effect for vitamin C increasing its effectiveness; prevent some bacterial and viral infections (Bidlack, 1998).

According to Brandt et al., (2011), who conducted a meta-analysis of the published comparative studies of the content of secondary metabolites in organic vs. conventional crops, organic ones contain 12% higher levels of favorable secondary metabolites than corresponding conventional fruits and vegetables.

In most studies comparing organic vs. conventional raw materials with respect to the content of secondary metabolites, the total amount of polyphenols is analysed, with no breakdown for individual compounds belonging to this group. To express the content of polyphenols in the plant, the conversion can be used, such as tannic acid (Carbonaro et al., 2002). The content of flavonoids or flavonols themselves can be expressed as equivalent amounts of quercetin (Rembiałkowska et al., 2003a and b; Young et al., 2005; Hallmann and Rembiałkowska, 2006). Moreover, Anttonen et al., (2006) analysed the organic and conventional strawberries with respect to individual substances: quercetin and kaempherol belonging to flavonols. As a separate group of polyphenolic compounds, the anthocyanins are tested in plant foods by many authors (Rembiałkowska et al., 2003 b; Rembiałkowska et al., 2004; Hallmann and Rembiałkowska, 2006; Tarozzi et al., 2006). Polyphenol content is compared by some authors as a dry matter of the product. However in most cases the content in the fresh plant product is analysed. Anyway, all of the analyzed studies - except one (Anttonen et al., 2006), which showed lower levels of one substance (kaempherol) in organic compared to conventional strawberries - indicate a significant advantage of fruits (apples, apple juice, stewed apple, peaches, pears, blackberries, strawberries, frozen strawberries, red oranges) derived from organic production (Weibel et al., 2000; Carbonaro and Mattera, 2001; Carbonaro et al., 2002; Asami et al., 2003; Rembiałkowska et al., 2003a; Rembiałkowska et al., 2004; Weibel et al., 2004; Rembiałkowska et al., 2006; Anttonen et al., 2006; Tarozzi et al., 2006). After averaging the results of the above research and application of a formula by Worthington (2001): (CONV-ORG) / ORG x 100% organic fruits contain on average 44.7% more polyphenols than conventional ones.

The studies performed on vegetables are also conducted with respect to the total polyphenol content, with no breakdown for individual substances. The comparative research shows that organic vegetables (frozen corn, tomatoes, Pac Choi Chinese cabbage, lettuce, red peppers and onions) contain significantly more polyphenols than conventional vegetables (Asami et al., 2003; Rembiałkowska et al., 2003b; Young et al., 2005; Hallmann et al., 2005; Hallmann and Rembiałkowska, 2006). After averaging the results of the above research and application of a formula by Worthington (2001): (CONV-ORG) / ORG x 100% organic vegetables contain on average 57.4% more polyphenols than conventional ones.

Carotenoids are another group of secondary metabolites of plants, characterized by strong antioxidative properties. They include over 600 pigments, which give the plants yellow, orange and red color. Carotenoids are also found in green leafy vegetables, but their color is masked by the green chlorophyll. The best-known carotenoid is beta-carotene found in many orange and yellow fruits and green leafy vegetables. Lycopene gives tomatoes intensive red color. Lutein and zeaxanthin make corn yellow. Carotenoids play an important role for human health, as they lower the blood cholesterol level, and thus favorably affect the heart. Moreover, they support the immune system - especially beta-carotene, which stimulates the increased number of lymphocytes. Carotenoids also exhibit antitumor activity, mainly thanks to its antioxidant properties (Stracke et al., 2008).

The comparative studies performed with respect to total carotenoid content in organic and conventional vegetables revealed the highest differences in case of pepper (Perez-Lopez et al., 2007). Slightly higher content of carotenoids (1.13%) was also found in organic tomatoes (Caris-Veyrat et al., 2004; Toor et al., 2006; Rickman Pieper and Barrett, 2009; Juroszek et al., 2009). The content of beta-carotene in organic carrots was higher, according to research by Abele (1987). By contrast Warman and Havard (1997) confirmed a lower content of beta-carotene in organic carrots. However, research by Caris-Veyrat et al., (2004) showed over 40% more beta-carotene in organic tomatoes.

The comparative studies conducted in the Organic Food Department of Warsaw University of Life Sciences confirmed significantly higher amount of beta-carotene in organic tomatoes and peppers (Rembiałkowska et al., 2003b; Hallmann et al., 2005; Hallmann et al., 2007), lutein in organic pepper (Hallmann et al., 2005; Hallmann et al., 2007) and total carotenoids in organic peppers (Hallmann et al., 2007; Hallmann et al., 2008; Hallmann and Rembiałkowska, 2008 a). However, higher lycopene content in organic material were found only in tomato juice (Hallmann and Rembiałkowska, 2008 b), whereas less lycopene in organic tomatoes and green peppers were found in comparison to conventional crops (Hallmann et al., 2005; Hallmann et al., 2007; Rembiałkowska et al., 2005; Hallmann and Rembiałkowska, 2007a and b; Hallmann and Rembiałkowska, 2008a).

The group of favourable antioxidants include also vitamin C, which performs fundamental metabolic functions in the human body. First of all it ensures the proper functioning of the immune system. Furthermore, it supports the biosynthesis of collagen, accelerates the process of wound healing and development of bones. In addition, it participates in the metabolism of fats, cholesterol and bile acids, regenerates vitamin E and other low molecular antioxidants such as glutathione and a has a stabilizing effect in relation to the flavonoids. Vitamin C exhibits bacteriostatic properties and even bactericidal activity against some pathogens. It supports the absorption of non-haem iron and is involved in the production of red blood cells. Vitamin C inhibits the formation of carcinogenic nitrosamines, thus it reduces the negative effect of nitrate intake (Mirvish, 1993).

Except two studies, which confirmed lower vitamin C content in organic frozen corn (Asami et al., 2003) and organic tomatoes (Rembiałkowska et al., 2003b), most of the results revealed that organic crops were characterized by a higher content of vitamin C: spinach (Schuphan, 1974; Vogtmann et al., 1984), celery (Schuphan, 1974; Leclerc et al., 1991), kale (Schuphan, 1974), cabbage (Rembiałkowska, 1998; Rembiałkowska, 2000), lettuce (Schuphan, 1974), leek (Lairon et al., 1984), potatoes (Schuphan, 1974; Petterson, 1978; Fischer and Richter, 1984; Rembiałkowska and Rutkowska, 1996; Rembiałkowska, 2000; Hajslova et al., 2005), Swiss chard (Moreira et al., 2003), onion (Hallmann and Rembiałkowska, 2006), tomatoes (Rembiałkowska et al., 2003b; Rembiałkowska et al., 2005; Hallmann et al., 2005), pepper (Hallmann et al., 2005; Hallmann et al., 2007), apples (Rembiałkowska et al., 2003a) and oranges (Rapisarda et al., 2005). After averaging the results of the above research and application of a formula by Worthington (2001): (CONV-ORG) / ORG x 100% organic materials contain on average 32.2% more vitamin C than conventional products. Recent meta-analysis of the various vitamins in vegetables and fruits showed that the organic raw materials contained on average 6.3% more vitamins than conventional raw materials, but the difference was not statistically significant (Hunter et al., 2011).

Summary of studies comparing the mineral content in organic vs. conventional vegetables (Worthington, 2001) indicates a higher content of minerals (iron, magnesium and phosphorus) in organic crops. According to the author, a possible reason of a higher content of mineral elements in organic raw materials is associated with a higher content of microorganisms in organically cultivated soil. The microorganisms generate compounds that support plants in introducing active substances adsorbed by soil minerals, making them more available for plant roots. Recent meta-analysis of mineral content showed that organic fruits and vegetables contain an average 5.5% more minerals than conventional ones (Hunter et al., 2011), and the difference was statistically significant. This was found with respect to boron, copper, magnesium, molybdenum, potassium, phosphorus, selenium, sodium and zinc. According to Lairon (2010), organic plant products contain higher concentrations of iron and magnesium, which can be explained with abovementioned factors.

There are several studies confirming the higher content of total sugars in organic fruits and vegetables, including carrots, beets, red beets, potatoes, spinach, kale, cherries, red currants and apples (Zadoks, 1989; Rembiałkowska, 1998; Rembiałkowska et al., 2004; Rembiałkowska, 2000; Hallmann and Rembiałkowska, 2006; Hallmann et al., 2007). The higher sugar content is associated with higher technological quality (for instance in case of sugar beet) and also with the higher sensory quality (taste). In research carried out both by consumers and by the trained panel, vegetables and fruits produced organically are often better evaluated in terms of their sensory properties (Rembiałkowska, 2000). Numerous studies based on the food preferences were also performed on rats. The results revealed better sensory properties of organic materials (Maeder et al., 1993; Velimirov, 2001; Velimirov, 2002). Rats that were fed both with organic and conventional food presented the tendency to choose organic carrots (81% of animals) and organic wheat (68%). Smaller differences were found in the choice of apples and red beets from organic farming, which, however, were also more likely to be selected by more than half (58%) of rats.

Several studies carried out so far (Rembiałkowska, 2000; Worthington, 2001) confirmed lower total amount of protein in organic crops compared to conventional. However, the protein quality (considered as the content of essential amino acids) were found to be higher in organic crops. According to Worthington (2001), nitrogen derived from each type of fertilizer affect the quantity and quality of proteins produced by plants. A large amount of nitrogen available to plants increases the production of proteins, and reduces carbohydrate production. Furthermore, proteins produced in response to high levels of nitrogen, present lower amounts of essential amino acids, e.g. lysine, and therefore represent lower nutritional value for consumers.

The higher technological value of organic plant products results from higher dry matter content, so that organic products perform better storage quality (Bulling, 1987; Rembiałkowska, 2000). Samaras (1978) confirmed that the main impact on the amount of weight loss after storage of vegetables is the type of fertilizer applied to them. All tested root vegetables (carrots, turnips, beets and potatoes), which were grown with organic fertilizer were characterized by much lower storage losses. The higher storage losses of vegetables grown with mineral fertilizer may be associated with a higher content of water absorbed by the plant, along with easily soluble mineral compounds. The average storage losses of crops grown with mineral fertilizers were 46.4% of the initial mass, whereas in case of crops grown with organic fertilization the losses were 28.9% (Samaras, 1978). Bulling (1987) made a set of studies comparing the differences in the storage losses between organic and conventional vegetables and fruits. Average values for the organic raw materials tested in 53 different studies were found to be 10% lower than for conventional crops. These properties are important both from nutritional and economic point of view. The hypothesis that plant materials from organic production is better to store was also confirmed by Benbrook (2005). Higher dry matter content of organic raw materials were observed in carrots (Velimirov, 2005), apples (Weibel, 2004; Rembiałkowska et al., 2004), potatoes (Rembiałkowska, 2000), strawberries (Reganold et al., 2010). However, Gąstoł et al., (2009) found lower dry matter content of organic apples and black currant than in conventional ones.

4. Animal products

Principles of organic animal husbandry refer to animal welfare (indoor farm density, access to open air, the presence of natural bedding, the possibility of movement), the nutrition (prohibition on synthetic feed additives) and rearing conditions (choice of breed, conditions of weaning and slaughter). Furthermore, organic livestock production is carried out without the use of antibiotics (except the situations, when the life of animal is endangered and there are no other therapeutic agents available), hormones, genetically modified organisms and their products. Organically reared animals can be fed only with organic materials.

A key factor determining the quality of animal products is the animal feed, which in case of organic agriculture involves the use of seasonal grazing and cutting down on feed concentrates, which is beneficial for the content of bioactive substances in meat and milk.

4.1. Meat

Meat derived from organic farming perform desirable nutritional properties, such as favorable ratios of fatty acids. This means the lower content of saturated and monounsaturated fatty acids, the higher content of polyunsaturated fatty acids, and a lower ratio of n-6 fatty acids to n-3 fatty acids. The meat produced organically exhibits also lower total fat content, which has been confirmed for: beef (Enser et al., 1998; Pastushenko et al., 2000), pork (Hansen et al., 2006; Bee et al., 2004; Nilzen et al., 2001; Kim et al., 2009), sheep (Fisher et al., 2000; Enser et al., 1998), lamb (Angood et al., 2007), poultry (Castellini et al., 2002). The studies conducted on poultry revealed different results, as higher content of saturated fatty acids was found in organic meat. However, it exhibited lower content of monounsaturated fatty acids and higher levelpolyunsaturated fatty acids. In turn, results obtained by Walshe et al., (2005) confirmed higher total fat content in organic beef, but comparable fatty acid composition in both types of meat. Research carried out on rabbit meat by Pla (2008) and Combes et al., (2003a) revealed a lower total fat content in meat derived from organically reared rabbits. However, Lebas et al., (2002) obtained opposite results.

Figure 3 below presents the comparison of fatty acid profile of *M. longissimus* muscle between organic and conventional pork derived from Korean black pigs (Kim et al., 2009).

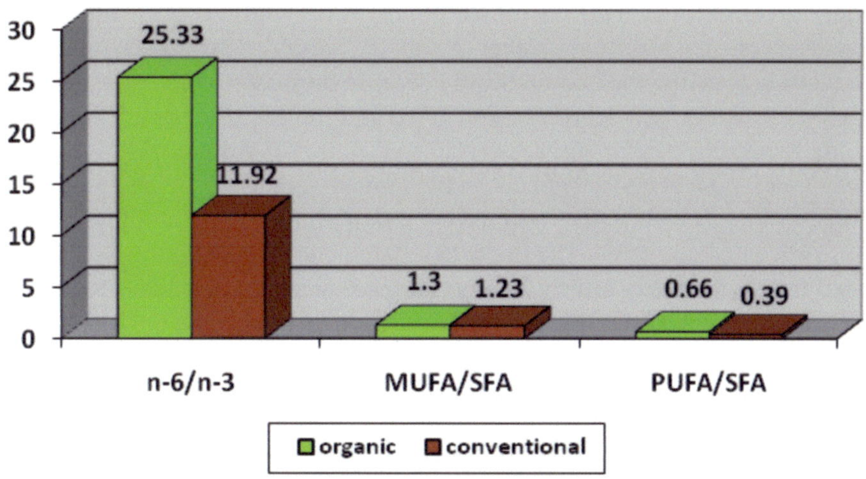

Figure 3. Fatty acid profile of organic and conventional pork from Korean black pigs (Kim et al., 2009)

Most of the studies confirm a higher content of intramuscular fat in organic meat, which was found in beef (Woodward and Fernandez, 1999), pork (Sundrum and Acosta, 2003; Millet et al., 2004), mutton (Fisher et al., 2000). The higher intramuscular fat content is associated with better sensory quality of meat from organic production. Only research done by Olsson et al., (2003) indicated a lower content of intramuscular fat and a lower lean body mass in organic pork.

As far as sensory quality is concerned, the darker meat color was identified in the case of organic pork (Kim et al., 2009; Millet et al., 2004) and sheep (Fisher et al., 2000). Research conducted by Fisher et al., (2000) found that organic lamb meat is preferred much more than conventional because of the sensory properties. Castellini et al., (2002) demonstrated with the sensory profile that the organic poultry is more juicy and acceptable than conventional. According to Combes et al., (2003b), the organic rabbit meat is softer than conventional. The sensory assessment done by Pla (2008) confirmed that organic rabbit meat exhibited more liver flavor and less anise and grass taste.

The adverse properties of organic meat include the lower carcass weight (lower daily weight gains), which has been confirmed for beef (Woodward and Fernandez, 1999), pork (Sundrum and Acosta, 2003; Hansen et al., 2006) and poultry (Castellini et al., 2002). However, study performed by Millet et al., (2004) indicated a higher weight gains of organic pigs in comparison to conventional ones.

Organic meat is also characterized by poor storage quality (high levels of TBARS), which was confirmed by analyses conducted on beef (Walshe et al., 2005), pork (Hansen et al., 2006; Nilzen et al., 2001), mutton (Fisher et al., 2000) and poultry (Castellini et al., 2002).

4.2. Milk

Cow's milk is very variable with respect to fat content. This fraction is formed in about 95%by triacylglycerols, which are composed of fatty acids whose chain length and degree of saturation determine the nutritional value of milk fat. Saturated fatty acids are considered as a factor adversely affecting the human health, because they contribute to the development of arteriosclerosis (Pfeuffer and Schrezenmeir, 2000) and increased levels of blood cholesterol, which leads to cardiovascular diseases (Haug et al, 2007). Among the unsaturated fatty acids, the n-3 ones pose beneficial effects on the human organism. N-3 acids affect positively the nervous system, as well as they reduce the risk of diabetes and cardiovascular diseases (Horrobin, 1993; Hu et al., 1999). The important parameter of milk quality is also the ratio of unsaturated fatty acids n-6:n-3. If the content of the first group of acids is too high, the risk of inflammation, thrombosis, and autoimmune symptoms is increased. The most important fatty acid among the n-3 acids is alpha-linolenic acid (LNA), while linoleic acid (LA) occurs in the largest quantities among the n-6 acids. As for monounsaturated fatty acids, oleic acid is the predominant one, amounting to about ¼ of the total weight of fatty acids. It supports the functioning of n-3 and n-6 acids, preventing them from oxidation, and lowers cholesterol and acts antineoplastic (Ip, 1997; Kris-Etherton et al., 1999; Mensink et al., 2003). A special place in the composition of cow's milk is conjugated linoleic acid (CLA). Cow's milk is the main source of the isomers of this compound in the human diet (Haug et al., 2004). The most important isomer (constituting about 90% of CLA) is *cis-9 trans-11*, preventing the development of cancer, heart disease and stimulating the immune system (Whigham et al., 2000). It is called rumenic acid because the rumen is the place of its synthesis from linoleic acid. Other CLA isomers (*trans-7 cis-9, trans-10 cis-12* and *trans-9 cis-11*) counteract obesity (by reducing fat and increasing muscle mass) and support the treatment of diabetes (Taylor and Zahradka, 2004). The content of CLA in milk fat is affected by a number of factors. First of all, it depends on the feed given to animals (Parodi, 1999), followed by seasonal variations (Parodi, 1977), the endogenous synthesis of trans-vaccenic acid (TVA) (Griinari et al., 2000) and oxidation of linoleic acid (LA) during processing (Ha et al., 1989).

The research comparing the quality of milk from different production systems is based on the analysis of particular differences in the composition of fatty acids (Molkentin and Giesemann, 2007; Butler et al., 2008). According to the results of Ellis et al., (2006) organic milk can be characterized with a significantly higher content of polyunsaturated fatty acids, including n-3 acids (the difference in comparison to conventional milk was over 60%). The ratio of n-6: n-3 was consequently lower, which is favorable from a health point of view. Moreover, the amount of polyunsaturated fatty acids relative to monounsaturated ones was found higher. The detailed results are presented in table 1. Similar conclusions were also drawn by Butler and Leifert (2009) who confirmed that the value of the ratio of n-6: n-3 in organically produced milk does not exceed 1.25, while in the conventional milk is above 2.5.

% FA	Conventional milk	Organic milk
SFA	67,25 ± 3,54	68,13 ± 3,51
MUFA	**27,63 ± 2,94**	**26,19 ± 3,01**
PUFA	**3,33 ± 0,66**	**3,89 ± 0,61**
total n-3	**0,66 ± 0,22**	**1,11 ± 0,25**
total n-6	1,68 ± 0,46	1,68 ± 0,44
TVA	1,75 ± 1,09	2,06 ± 0,96
CLA	0,58 ± 0,34	0,65 ± 0,28

Table 1. Differences in fatty acid composition between organic and conventional milk (Ellis et al., 2006)

Qualitative changes in milk, resulting from the application of ecological production system, can be also identified in the concentration of CLA (Bergamo et al., 2003; Szente et al., 2006). A study by Butler et al., (2008) revealed that its amount may be higher by up to 60% compared to the content in the conventional milk. Research byJahreis et al., (1996) confirms that the organic production of milk contributes to increased concentrations of CLA, TVA and LNA. This was also indicated by research by Chin et al., (1992), Lin et al., (1995), Prandini et al., (2001), particularly in relation to CLA content in cow's milk and buffalo milk. However, few studies showed no difference in the amount of CLA between milk from both production systems (Ellis et al., 2006; Toledo et al., 2002).

Antioxidants, especially vitamin E and carotenoids, are another advantage for the consumption of organically produced milk. Their content was found higher in milk from cows from organic husbandry and this corresponds to the fact that the feeding of such cattle is based on green forage pasture (Nielsen et al., 2004; Butler et al., 2008). This has been also confirmed by the research conducted within the project QLIF (Quality Low Input Food). The level of antioxidants in organic milk was almost double compared to conventional milk (QLIF, 2008).

Palupi et al., (2012) carried out a meta-analysis of comparative studies related to the nutritional quality of organic and conventional dairy products. The authors' approach used the Hedges' d effect size method with regard to the results obtained by various authors in the last three years. The meta-analysis confirmed, that compared to conventional dairy products, organic ones exhibit significantly higher content of protein, alpha-linolenic acid, conjugated linoleic acid, transvaccenic acid, docosapentanoic acid, eicosapentanoic acid and the total n-3 fatty acids. Furthermore, the n-3:n-6 ratio was found to be significantly higher in organically produced dairy products (0,42 vs. 0,23).

Organic production implies the abandonment of the use of mineral supplements, making the content of these components generally higher in conventionally produced milk. This has been confirmed by Coonan et al., (2002), who found the deficiencies of copper, selenium, zinc, iodine and molybdenum in the organic milk. Kuusela and Okker (2007) explain this as a result of a low content of trace elements in soil within organic farms. The use of synthetic fertilizers, which increase the concentration of macro- and microelements in soil are not permitted in organic farming. The crops, which have grown within such soil, are as a consequence a poor feed for animals with respect to these components, which contributes to their deficiency in milk. However, few studies showed a higher calcium content in organically produced milk (Lund and Algers, 2003; Zadoks, 1989).

Apart from the abovementioned benefits milk of organic production has one more advantage over the conventional milk. This is a prohibition on the use of antibiotics, which are often routinely given by conventional farmers to farm animals for the purposes of prevention. In the certified organic farms such practices are prohibited. The issue of the impact of antibiotics in conventionally fed cows on the resistance of the human body to these antibiotics is still a topic of discussion. The use of synthetic hormones and genetically modified feed ingredients is also not allowed in organic system. For this reason, the residues listed above, which are frequently detected in conventional dairy products, are negligible in milk from organic production. Research conducted by USDA (United States Department of Agriculture) confirmed this hypothesis by detecting the presence of pyretroid pesticides in 27% of conventional milk samples. Among the organic samples, only one contained a low level of these substances, while others were completely free of these contaminants (Benbrook, 2005). The analysis of heavy metals in both types of milk showed no differences between the samples, detecting low contamination of all samples (Gabryszuk et al., 2008).

Sensory quality assessments of organic and conventional milk are very rare and so far inconclusive. Research by Zadoks (1989) showed greater acceptability of conventional milk among consumers. The predominant factor responsible for this result was the peculiar smell of cow's milk, much more intense in the case of organic milk. Today's consumers are not used to such properties, preferring generally available in the market milk with a neutral smell. Croissant et al., (2007) found that consumers felt more grassy and animal smell in milk derived from organic production compared to typical conventional milk, but only when the temperature of milk was 15°C. No differences between milk from both systems were found at a temperature of milk of 7°C. The authors concluded that there are clear differences between the smell and quality of milk from organic and conventional systems, but this has no effect on consumer acceptance.

5. Conclusions

The favorable high nutritional value of food depends not only on the appropriate content of compounds necessary for the proper functioning of the human body and the low content of harmful substances. According to studies cited here, the nutrient content in plant raw materials in most cases is higher when they come from organic farming. This includes the compounds belonging to the desirable antioxidants: vitamin C, phenolic compounds, carotenoids, as well as sugars and dry matter. The latter two components both contribute to higher technological value and reduction of storage losses. Furthermore, they significantly increase the palatability of organic fruits and vegetables. As a result, the flavor of organic products may be more intense compared to conventional materials, so that consumers evaluate the taste of organic materials as more typical, characteristic of the plant, which is also confirmed by preference tests performed on animals.

In terms of pesticides and nitrates from the consumer point of view raw materials from organic production are certainly safer than conventional. The level of mycotoxins is dependent not only on the production system, but is also affected by storage and weather conditions. Studies show that there are no significant differences in the content of cereals with mycotoxins between organic and conventional products.

Meat derived from organically reared animals exhibit positive quality characteristics, such as favorable ratios of fatty acids and low total fat content. Organic meat is also better evaluated according to their sensory qualities, which is associated with a higher intramuscular fat content. The unfavorable properties of organic meat include lower carcass weight (lower daily weight gain), and inferior storage quality (high levels of TBARS).

Milk from organic production is characterized by a favorable fatty acid composition (including a high content of CLA), high levels of vitamins and antioxidants, acting an important part health-oriented prevention. However, due to the ban on the use of mineral supplements and fertilizers in organic farming, milk from organic production may be characterized by the deficiency of some macro- and micronutrients. Moreover, milk from organically reared animals can be worse evaluated by consumers because of the specific organoleptic characteristics, especially the smell.

According to Dangour et al., (2010) and Huber et al., (2011), the higher nutritional value of organic foodstuffs cannot be simply considered as an evidence, that consumption of organic food contributes to the improvement of consumers' health. Based on the research carried out so far, no clear relationship between nutritional value and health effects can be defined. Evidence for such effects are still lacking, therefore more developed studies are needed to determine the nutrition-related health effects that result from the consumption of organic products.

Acknowledgements

We are very grateful to dr Johannes Kahl from University of Kassel, Dep. Organic Food Quality and Food Culture for his careful pre-review and amendments.

Author details

Ewa Rembiałkowska[1,2], Aneta Załęcka[1,2], Maciej Badowski[1] and Angelika Ploeger[3,2]

1 Warsaw University of Life Sciences, Faculty of Human Nutrition and Consumer Sciences, Poland

2 International Organic FQH Research Association

3 Kassel University, Department of Organic Food Quality and Food Culture, Germany

References

[1] Abele, U. (1987). Produktqualität und Düngung- mineralisch, organisch, biologisch-dynamisch. Angewendte Wissenschaft (Schriftenreihe des Bundesministers für Ernährung, Landwirtschaft und Forsten), Heft 345.

[2] AFSCA-FAVV,(2001). Chemical safety of organically produced foodstuffs. Report from the scientific committee of the Belgian federal agency for the safety of the food chain (AFSCA-FAVV), Brussels.

[3] Angood, K. M., Wood, J. D., Nute, G. R., Whittington, F. M., Hughes, S. I., & Sheard, P. R. (2008). A comparison of organic and conventionally-produced lamb purchased from three major UK supermarkets: Price, eating quality and fatty acid composition. Meat Science , 78, 176-184.

[4] Anttonen, M. J., Hoppula, K. I., Nestby, R., Verheul, M. J., & Karjalainen, R. O. (2006). Influence of fertilization, mulch color, early forcing, fruit order, planting date, shading, growing environment, and genotype on the contents of selected phenolics in strawberry (Fragaria × ananassaDuch.) fruits. J Agric Food Chem, , 54, 2614-2620.

[5] Asami, D. K., Hong, Y., , J., Barrett, D. M., & Mitchell, A. E. (2003). Comparison of the Total Phenolic and Ascorbic Acid Content of Freeze-Dried and Air-Dried Marionberry, Strawberry, and Corn Grown Using Conventional, Organic, and Sustainable Agricultural Practices. J. Agric. Food Chem., , 51, 1237-1241.

[6] Aubert, C. (1987). Pollution du lait maternel, une enquete de Terre vivante. Les Quatre Saisons du Jardinage, , 42, 33-39.

[7] Baker, B. P., Benbrook, C. M., Groth, E., & Benbrook, K. L. (2002). Pesticide residues in conventional, integrated pest management (IPM)-grown and organic foods: insights from three US data sets. Food Additives and Contaminants, , 19, 427-446.

[8] Bee, G., Guex, G., & Herzog, W. (2004). Free-range rearing of pigs during the winter: Adaptations in muscle fiber characteristics and effects on adipose tissue composition and meat quality traits. J. Anim. Sci. , 82, 1206-1218.

[9] Benbrook, C. M. (2005). FAQS on Pesticides in Milk. Organic Center.Calculated from USDA's Pesticide Data Program.

[10] Bergamo, P., Fedele, E., Iannibeli, L., & Marzillo, G. (2003). Fat-soluble vitamins contents and fatty acid composition in organic and conventional Italian dairy products. Food Chemistry , 82, 625-631.

[11] Bidlack, W. W. (1998). Functional Foods. Biochemical and Processing Aspects. G. Mazza, red. Lancaster, PA: Technomic Publishing Co., Inc., , 437.

[12] BMA,(1992). The BMA guide to pesticides, chemicals and health. Report of science and education. British Medical Association, UK.

[13] Brandt, K., & Molgaard, J. P. (2001). Organic agriculture: does it enhance or reduce the nutritional value of plant foods? J. Sci. Food Agric. , 81, 924-931.

[14] Brandt, K., Leifert, C., Sanderson, R., & Seal, C. J. (2011). Agroecosystem Management and Nutritional Quality of Plant Foods: The Case of Organic Fruits and Vegetables. Critical Reviews in Plant Sciences , 30, 177-197.

[15] Bulling, W. (1987). Qualitätsvergleich von "biologisch" und "konventionell" erzeugten Feldfruchten. Regierungspräsidium, Stuttgart.

[16] Butler, G., & Leifert, C. (2009). Effect of organic production methods on product quality and animal health and welfare; why are there differences? Proceedings of the conference on Improvement of quality of animal products obtained in sustainable production systems with special reference to bioactive components and their benefit for human health, May 2009, Jastrzębiec, 88-93., 14-15.

[17] Butler, G., Nielsen, J. H., Slots, T., Seal, C., Eyre, M. D., Sanderson, R., & Leifert, C. (2008). Fatty acid and fat-soluble antioxidant concentrations in milk from high- and low-input conventional and organic systems: seasonal variation. Journal of the Science of Food and Agriculture , 88, 1431-1441.

[18] Carbonaro, M., & Mattera, M. (2001). Polyphenoloxidase activity and polyphenol levels in organically and conventionally grown peach (Prunuspersica L., cv. Regina bianca) and pear (Pyruscommunis L., cv. Williams). Food Chemistry, , 72, 419-424.

[19] Carbonaro, M., Mattera, M., Nicoli, S., Bergamo, P., & Cappelloni, M. (2002). Modulation of antioxidant compounds in organic vs. conventional fruit (Peach, Prunuspersica L, and Pear, Pyruscommunis L.). J Agric Food Chem , 50, 5458-5462.

[20] Caris-Veyrat, C., Amiot, M. J., Tyssandier, V., Grasselly, D., Buret, M., Mikolajczak, M., Guilland, J. C., Bouteloup-Demange, C., & Borel, P. (2004). Influence of organic versus conventional agricultural practice on the antioxidant microconstituent content of tomatoes and derived purees; consequences on antioxidant plasma status in humans. J Agric Food Chem, , 52, 6503-6509.

[21] Castellini, C., Mugnai, C., & Dal, Bosco. A. (2002). Effect of organic production system on broiler carcass and meat quality. Meat Sci. , 60, 219-225.

[22] Chin, S. F., Liu, W., Storkson, J. M., Ha, Y. L., & Pariza, M. W. (1992). Dietary sources of conjugated dienoic isomers of linoleic acid, a newly recognized class of anticarcinogens. Journal of Food Composition and Analysis, , 5, 185-197.

[23] Combes, S., Lebas, F., Juin, H., Lebreton, L., Martin, T., Jehl, N., Cauquil, L., Darche, B. i., & Corboeuf, M. A. (2003b). Comparaison lapin " Bio "/ lapin standard : Analyses sensorielles et tendretemecanique de la viande. 10emes Journées de la Recherche Cunicole, Paris, , 137-140.

[24] Combes, S., Lebas, F., Lebreton, L., Martin, T., Jehl, N., Cauquil, L., Darche, B., & Corboeuf, M. A. (2003a). Comparison lapin " Bio "/ lapin standard : Caractéristique des carcasses et composition chimique de 6 muscles de la cuisse. Proc. 10emes Journées de la Recherche Cunicole, Paris, , 133-136.

[25] Coonan, C., Freestone-Smith, C., Allen, J., & Wilde, D. (2002). Determination of the major mineral and trace element balance of dairy cows in organic production systems. W: Proceeding of Organic Meat and Milk from Ruminants (Red.Kyriazakis, Zervas), Athens, October 4-6, 2002, EAAP Publication, , 106

[26] Croissant, A. E., Washburn, S. P., Dean, L. L., & Drake, M. A. (2007). Chemical Properties and Consumer Perception of Fluid Milk from Conventional and Pasture-Based Production Systems. Journal of Dairy Science, , 90(11), 4942-4953.

[27] Curl, C. L., Fenske, R. A., & Elgethun, K. (2003). Organophosphate pesticide exposure of urban and suburban preschool children with organic and conventional diets. Environ Health Perspect. , 111, 377-382.

[28] Dangour, A. D., Lock, K., Hayter, A., Aikenhead, A., Allen, E., & Uauy, R. (2010). Nutrition-related health effects of organic foods:systematic review. Am J Clin Nutr , 92, 203-210.

[29] Di Renzo, L., Di Pierro, D., Bigioni, M., Sodi, V., Galvano, F., & Cianci, R. (2007). Is antioxidant plasma status in humans a consequence of the antioxidant food content influence? European review for medical and pharmacological Sciences, , 185-192.

[30] EFSA Journal,(2010). Scientific Report of EFSA, 2008 Annual Report on Pesticide Residues according to Article 32 of Regulation (EC) European Food Safety Authority. European Food Safety Authority (EFSA), Parma, Italy, 8(6): 1646.(396)

[31] EFSA Scientific Report,(2009). Annual Report on Pesticide Residues according to Article 32 of Regulation (EC) Prepared by Pesticides Unit (PRAPeR) of EFSA (Question No EFSA-Q-2008-714), 305, 1-106.(396)

[32] Ellis, K. A., Innocent, G. T., Grove-White, D., Cripps, P., Mc Lean, W. G., Howard, C. V., & Mihm, M. (2006). Comparing the fatty acid composition of organic and conventional milk. Journal of Dairy Science , 89, 1938-1950.

[33] Enser, M., Hallett, K. G., Hewett, B., Fursey, G. A. J., Wood, J. D., & Harrington, G. (1998). Fatty acid content and composition of UK beef and lamb muscle in relation to production system and implications for human nutrition. Meat Sci. , 49, 329-341.

[34] Fischer, A., & Richter, C. (1984). Influence of organic and mineral fertilizers on yield and quality of potatoes. (W:) The Importance of Biological Agriculture in a World of Diminishing Resources (Red.Vogtmann H, Boehncke E, Fricke I). Witzenhausen.VerlagsgruppeWeiland, 1984: 236 248.

[35] Fisher, A. V., Enser, M., Richardson, R. I., Wood, J. D., Nute, G. R., Kurt, E., Sinclair, L. A., & Wilkinson, R. G. (2000). Fatty acid composition and eating quality of lamb types derived from four diverse breedx production system. Meat Sci. , 55, 141-147.

[36] Gabryszuk, M., Słoniewski, K., & Sakowski, T. (2008). Macro- and microelements in milk and hair of cows from conventional vs. organic farms. Animal Science Papers and Reports 26 (3), 199-209.

[37] Gąstoł, M., Domagała-Świątkiewicz, I., & Krośniak, M. (2009). Właściwości prozdrowotne produktów i przetworów uzyskanych metodą ekologiczną i konwencjonalną-analiza porównawcza. Uniwersytet Rolniczy im. Hugona Kołłątaja w Krakowie, , 30-32.

[38] Gnusowski, B., & Nowacka, A. (2007). Pozostałości środków ochrony roślin w polskich płodach rolnych pochodzących z różnych systemów gospodarowania. FragmentaAgronomica 3 (95), 121-125.

[39] Gottschalk, C., Barthel, J., Engelhardt, G., Bauer, J., & Meyer, K. (2007). Occurrence of type A trichothecenes in conventionally and organically produced oats and oat products. Mol.Nutr. FoodRes., , 51, 1547-1553.

[40] Griinari, J. M., Corl, B. A., Lacy, S. H., Chouinard, P. Y., Nurmela, K. V. V., & Bauman, D. E. (2000). Conjugated linoleic acid is synthesized endogenously in lactating dairy cows by Δ9-desaturase. Journal of Nutrition, , 130, 2285-2291.

[41] Guadagnin, S. G., Rath, S., & Reyes, F. G. R. (2005). Evaluation of the nitrate content in leaf vegetables produced through different agricultural systems. Food Additives and Contaminants, , 22(12), 1203-1208.

[42] Ha, Y. L., Grimm, N. K., & Pariza, M. W. (1989). Newly recognized anticarcinogenic fatty acids: identification and quantification in natural and processed cheese. Journal of Agricultural and Food Chemistry, , 37, 75-81.

[43] Hajslova, J., Schulzova, V., Slanina, P., Janne, K., Hellenas, K. E., & Andersson, Ch. (2005). Quality of organically and conventionally grown potatoes: Four-year study of micronutrients, metals, secondary metabolites, enzymic browning and organoleptic properties. Food Addit. Contam. , 22, 514-534.

[44] Hallmann, E., & Rembiałkowska, E. (2006). Zawartość związków antyoksydacyjnych w wybranych odmianach cebuli z produkcji ekologicznej i konwencjonalnej. Journal of Research and Applications in Agricultural Engineering 51 (2), 42- 46.

[45] Hallmann, E., & Rembiałkowska, E. (2007a). Zawartość związków bioaktywnych w owocach papryki z uprawy ekologicznej i konwencjonalnej. ŻywienieCzłowieka i Metabolizm, XXXIV, , 538-543.

[46] Hallmann, E., & Rembiałkowska, E. (2007b). Comparison of the nutritive quality of tomato fruits from organic and conventional production in Poland. Proceedings of the 3rd International Congress of the European Integrated Project Quality Low Input Food (QLIF) (Red. U. Niggli i in.), University of Hohenheim, Germany, March 20-23: 131-135

[47] Hallmann, E., & Rembiałkowska, E. (2008a). The content of selected antioxidant compounds in bell pepper varieties from organic and conventional cultivationbefore and after freezing process. Proceedings of the Second Scientific Conference of the International Society of Organic Agriculture Research (ISOFAR) (Red.D. Neuhoff I in.).Modena, 18-20 June, , 2

[48] Hallmann, E., & Rembiałkowska, E. (2008b). Ocena wartości odżywczej i sensorycznej pomidorówoaz soku pomidorowego z produkcji ekologicznej i konwencjonalnej. Journal of Research and Applications in Agricultural Engineering, 53/ , 3, 88-95.

[49] Hallmann, E., Rembiałkowska, E., & Kaproń, L. (2005). Zawartość związków bioaktywnych w pomidorach i papryce z uprawy ekologicznej i konwencjonalnej. Wybrane zagadnienia ekologiczne we współczesnym rolnictwie. Monografia, PIMR, Poznań, tom , 2, 258-263.

[50] Hallmann, E., Rembiałkowska, E., Szafirowska, A., & Grudzień, K. (2007). Znaczenie surowców z produkcji ekologicznej w profilaktyce zdrowotnej na przykładzie papryki z uprawy ekologicznej. Roczniki PZH 2007, 58/, 1, 77-82.

[51] Hallmann, E., Sikora, M., & Rembiałkowska, E. (2008). Porównanie zawartości związków przeciwutleniających w owocach papryki świeżej i mrożonej pochodzącej z uprawy ekologicznej i konwencjonalnej. PostępyTechnikiPrzetwórstwaSpożywczego, 18/, 1, 30-33.

[52] Hansen, L. L., Cludi-Magnussen, C., Jensen, S. K., & Andersen, H. J. (2006). Effect of organic production system on performance and meat quality. Meat Sci. , 74, 605-615.

[53] Hassold-Piezunka, N. (2003). Eignung des Chroma-Boden-Tests zur Bestimmung von Kompostqualität und Rottegrad. Pracadoktorska.Universität Oldenburg.

[54] Haug, A., Hostmark, A. T. i., & Harstad, O. M. (2007). Bovine milk in human nutrition-a review. Lipids in Health and Disease 6, 25 (www.lipidworld.com/content/6/I/25).

[55] Haug, A., Taugbol, O., Olsen, E. S., Biong, A. S., & Harstad, O. M. (2004). Milk fat in human nutrition. Studies in dairy cows with special reference to CLA. Animal Science Papers and Reports, , 22(3)

[56] Horrobin, D. F. (1993). Fatty acid metabolism in health and disease: the role of delta-desaturase. American Journal of Clinical Nutrition 57, 732S-736S., 6.

[57] Howard, V. (2005). Pesticides and Health. W: A lecture at the Congress: "Organic Farming, Food Quality and Human Health". January 2005, Newcastle, UK., 5-6.

[58] Hu, F. B., Stampfer, M. J., Manson, J. E., Rimm, E. B., Wolk, A., Colditz, G. A., Hennekens, C. H., & Willett, W. C. (1999). Dietary intake of {alpha}-linolenic acid and risk of fatal ischemic heart disease among women. American Journal of Clinical Nutrition 69(5), 890- 897.

[59] Huber, M., Rembiałkowska, E., Średnicka, D., Bügel, S., & van de Vijver, L. P. L. (2011). Organic food and impact on human health: Assessing the status quo and prospects of research. Wageningen Journal of Life Sciences , 58, 103-109.

[60] Hunter, D., Foster, M., Mc Arthur, J. O., Ojha, R., Petocz, P., & Samman, S. (2011). Evaluation of the Micronutrient Composition of Plant Foods produced by Organic and Conventional Agricultural Methods. Critical Reviews In Food Science and Nutrition, , 51, 571-582.

[61] Ip, C. (1997). Review of the effects of trans fatty acids, oleic acid, n-3 polyunsaturated fatty acids, and conjugated linoleic acid on mammary carcinogenesis in animals. American Journal of Clinical Nutrition 66, 1523S-1529S.

[62] Jahreis, G., Fritsche, J., & Steinhart, H. (1996). Monthly variations of milk composition with special regards to fatty acids depending on season and farm management systems-conventional versus ecological. Fett/Lipid, , 98, 365-369.

[63] Jestoi, M., Somma, M. C., Kouva, M., Veijalainen, P., Rizzo, A., Ritieni, A., & Peltonen, K. (2004). Levels of mycotoxins and sample cytotoxicity of selected organic and conventional grain-based products purchased from Finnish and Italian markets. Mol.Nutr. FoodRes, , 48, 299-307.

[64] Juroszek, P., Lumpkin, H. M., Yang, R., , Y., Ledesma, D. R., , C., & , H. (2009). Fruit Quality and Bioactive Compounds with Antioxidant Activity of Tomatoes Grown On-Farm: Comparison of Organic and Conventional Management Systems. Journal of the Agricultural and Food Chemistry, , 57, 1188-1194.

[65] Kahl, J., Busscher, N., & Ploeger, A. (2010). Questions on the Validation of Holistic Methods of Testing Organic Food Quality. Biological Agriculture and Horticulture, , 27, 81-94.

[66] Kim, D. H., Seong, P. N., Cho, S. H., Kim, J. H., Lee, J. M., Jo, C., & Lim, D. G. (2009). Fatty acid composition and meat quality traits of organically reared Korean native black pigs. Livestock Science , 120(2009), 96-102.

[67] Kouba, M. (2003). Quality of organic animal products. Livestock Production Science, , 80, 33-40.

[68] Kris-Etherton, P. M., Pearson, T. A., Wan, Y., Hargrove, R. L., Moriarty, K., Fishell, V., & Etherton, T. D. (1999). High-monounsaturated fatty acid diets lower both plasma cholesterol and triacylglycerol concentrations. American Journal of Clinical Nutrition , 70, 1009-15.

[69] Kummeling, I., Thijs, C., Huber, M., van de Vijver, L. P., Snijders, B. E., Penders, J., Stelma, F., van Ree, R., van den, Brandt. P. A., & Dagnelie, P. C. (2008). Consumption of organic foods and risk of atopic disease during the first 2 years of life in the Netherlands. Br. J. Nutr. 99(3), 598-605.

[70] Kuusela, E. i., & Okker, L. (2007). Influence of organic practices on selenium concentration of tank milk-a farm study. Journal of Animal and Feed Sciences 16, Suppl. I, , 97-101.

[71] Lairon, D., Termine, E., Gauthier, S., Trouilloud, M., Lafont, H., Hauton, J., & Ch, . (1984). Effects of Organic and Mineral Fertilization on the Contents of Vegetables in Minerals, Vitamin C and Nitrates, W: The Importance of Biological Agriculture in a World of Diminishing Resources. Proc. (Red.H.Vogtmann i in.), 5th IFOAM Conference, Verlagsgruppe, Witzenhausen.

[72] Lairon, D., & 201, . (2010). Nutritional quality and safety of organic food.A review.Agron Sustain Dev , 30, 33-41.

[73] Lebas, F., Lebreton, L., & Martin, T. (2002). Statistics on organic production of rabbits on grassland. Cuniculture , 164, 74-80.

[74] Leclerc, J., Miller, M. L., Joliet, E., & Rocquelin, G. (1991). Vitamin and Mineral Contents of Carrotand Celeriac Grown under Mineral or Organic Fertilization, Biological Agriculture and Horticulture, , 7, 339-348.

[75] Leszczyńska, T. (1996). Azotany i azotyny w warzywach pochodzących z upraw konwencjonalnych i ekologicznych, Bromat. ChemiaToksykol., , 29(3), 289-293.

[76] Lin, H., Boylston, T. D., Chang, M. J., Luedcke, L. O., & Shultz, T. D. (1995). Survey of the conjugated linoleic acid contents of dairy products. Journal of Dairy Science, , 78, 2358-2365.

[77] Lund, V., Algers, B., & 200, . (2003). Research on animal health and welfare in organic farming- a literature review.Livestock Production Science. , 80, 55-68.

[78] Lundegardh, B., & Martensson, A. (2003). Organically Produced Plant Food Evidence of Health Benefits. Soil and Plant Sci., , 53, 3-15.

[79] Maeder, P., Hahn, D., Dubois, D., Gunst, L., Alföldi, T., Bergmann, H., Oehme, M., Amado, R., Schneider, H., Graf, U., Velimirov, A., Fließbach, A., & Niggli, U. (2007). Wheat quality in organic and conventional farming: results of a 21 year field experiment, J. Sci. Food Agric. , 87, 1826-1835.

[80] Maeder, P., Pfiffner, L., Niggli, U., Balzer, U., Balzer, F., Plochberger, K., Velimirov, A., & Besson-M, J. (1993). Effect of three farming systems (bio-dynamic, bio-organic, conventional) on yield and quality of beetroot (Beta vulgaris L. var. esculenta L.) in a seven year crop rotation. Acta Hor., , 339, 10-31.

[81] Mensink, R. P., Zock, P. L., Kester, A. D. i., & Katan, M. B. (2003). Effects of dietary fatty acids and carbohydrates on the ratio of serum total to HDL cholesterol and on serum lipids and apolipoproteins: a meta-analysis of 60 controlled trials. American Journal of Clinical Nutrition , 77, 1146-55.

[82] Millet, S., Hesta, M., Seynaeve, M., Ongenae, E., De Smet, S., Debraekeleer, J. i., & Janssens, G. P. J. (2004). Performance, meat and carcass traits of fattening pigs with organic versus conventional hausing and nutrition. Livest. Prod. Sci. , 87, 109-119.

[83] Mirvish, S. S. (1993). Vitamin C inhibition of N-nitroso compounds formation. Am. J. Clin. Nutr. , 57, 598-599.

[84] Molkentin, J., & Giesemann, A. (2007). Differentiation of organically and conventionally produced milk by stable isotope and fatty acid analysis. Analytical and Bioanalytical Chemistry 388(1), 297-305.

[85] Moreira, M. R., Roura, S. I., & Del Valle, C. E. (2003). Quality of Swiss chard produced by conventional and organic methods. Lebensm.-Wiss. U.-Technol., , 36, 135-141.

[86] Nielsen, J. H., Lund-Nielsen, T., & Skibsted, L. (2004). Higher antioxidant content in organic milk than in conventional milk due to feeding strategy. DARCOFenews, Newsletter from Danish Research Centre for Organic Farming, 3 (http://www.darcof.dk/enews/sep04/milk.html).

[87] Nilzen, V., Babol, J., Dutta, P. C., Lundeheim, N., Enfält, A. C., & Lundstrom, K. (2001). Free range rearing of pigs with access to pasture grazing- effect on fatty acid composition and lipid oxidation products. Meat Sci. , 58, 267-275.

[88] Olsson, V., Andersson, K., Hansson, I., & Lundström, K. (2003). Differences in meat quality between organically and conventionally produced pigs. Meat Sci. 64 (3), 287-297.

[89] Palupi, E., Jayanegara, A., Ploeger, A., & Kahl, J. (2012). Comparison of nutritional quality between conventional and organic dairy products: a meta-analysis. J Sci Food Agric 2012.

[90] Parodi, P. W. (1977). Conjugated octadecadienoic acids of milk fat. Journal of Dairy Science, , 60, 1550-1553.

[91] Parodi, P. W. (1999). Conjugated linoleic acid and other anticarcinogenic agents of bovine milk fat. Journal of Dairy Science, , 82, 1339-1349.

[92] Pastushenko, V., Matthes, H., , D., Hein, T., & Holzer, Z. (2000). Impact of cattle grazing on meat fatty acid composition in relation to human health. Proc. th IFOAM Sci. Conf., Basel, s. 693., 13.

[93] Perez-Lopez, A. J., Fortea, M. I., Del Amor, F. M., Serrano-Martinez, A., & Nunez-Delicado, E. (2007). Influence of agricultural practices on the quality of sweet pepper fruits as affected by the maturity stage. J Sci Food and Agric, , 87, 2075-2080.

[94] Petterson, B. D. (1978). A Comparison between the Conventional and Biodynamic Farming Systems as Indicated by Yields and Quality, W: International IFOAM Conference- Towards a Sustainable Agriculture- Sissach.

[95] Pfeuffer, M., & Schrezenmeir, J. (2000). Bioactive substances in milk with properties decreasing risk of cardiovascular disease. British Journal of Nutrition 84 (1), 155-159.

[96] Pla, M. (2008). A comparison of the carcass traits and meat quality of conventionally and organically produced rabbits. Livestock Science , 115, 1-12.

[97] Prandini, A., Geromin, D., Conti, F., Masoero, F., Piva, A., & Piva, G. (2001). Survey on the level of conjugated linoleic acid in dairy products. Italian Journal of Food Science, , 13, 243-253.

[98] Pussemier, L., Larondelle, Y., Peteghem, C., & Huyghebaert, A. (2006). Chemical safety of conventionally and organically produced food stuffs: a tentative comparison under Belgian conditions. Food control, , 6, 14-21.

[99] QLIF (Quality Low Input Food),. (2008). www.qlif.org.

[100] Rapisarda, P., Calabretta, M. L., Romano, G., & Intrigliolo, F. (2005). Nitrogen Metabolism Components as a Tool To Discriminate between Organic and Conventional Citrus Fruits. J. Agric. Food Chem., 2005, 53 (7), 2664-2669.

[101] Reganold, J., Andrews, P., Reeve, J., Carpenter-Boggs, L., Schadt, Ch., Alldredge, R., Ross, C., Davies, N., & Zhou, J. (2010). Fruit and Soil Quality of Organic and Conventional strawberry Agroecosystems. PlusOne, 5/ , 9, 123-137.

[102] Rembiałkowska, E. (1998). Badania porównawcze jakości zdrowotnej i odżywczej marchwi i białej kapusty z gospodarstw ekologicznych i konwencjonalnych. Rocz. AR Pozn. CCCIV, Ogrod., , 27, 257-266.

[103] Rembiałkowska, E. (2000). Zdrowotna i sensoryczna jakość ziemniaków oraz wybranych warzyw z gospodarstw ekologicznych. Fundacja Rozwój SGGW, Warszawa.

[104] Rembiałkowska, E., Adamczyk, M., & Hallmann, E. (2003a). Jakość sensoryczna i wybrane cechy jakości odżywczej jabłek z produkcji ekologicznej i konwencjonalnej. Bromat.Chem. Toksykol., , 36, 33-40.

[105] Rembiałkowska, E., Adamczyk, M., & Hallmann, E. (2004). Porównanie wybranych cech wartości odżywczej jabłek z produkcji ekologicznej i konwencjonalnej, Bromat. Chem. Toksykol- Suplement, , 201-207.

[106] Rembiałkowska, E., Hallmann, E., Adamczyk, M., Lipowski, J., Jasińska, U., & Owczarek, L. (2006). Wpływ procesów technologicznych na zawartość polifenoli ogółem oraz potencjał przeciwutleniający przetworów (soku i kremogenu) uzyskanych z jabłek pochodzących z produkcji ekologicznej i konwencjonalnej. Żywność, Technologia Jakość, 1(46), Suplement, , 121-126.

[107] Rembiałkowska, E., Hallmann, E., & Szafirowska, A. (2005). Nutritive quality of tomato fruits from organic and conventional cultivation. Culinary Arts and Sciences V. Global and National Perspectives. (Red. Edwards, J.S.A., Kowrygo, B., Rejman, K.). , 193-202.

[108] Rembiałkowska, E., Hallmann, E., & Wasiak-Zys, G. (2003b). Jakość odżywcza i sensoryczna pomidorów z uprawy ekologicznej i konwencjonalnej. Żywienie Człowieka i Metabolizm, , 30, 893-899.

[109] Rembiałkowska, E., & Rutkowska, B. (1996). Comparison of sensory, nutritional and storage quality of potatoes from ecological and conventional farms. W: Proc. of the 5th International Conf. "Quality for European Integration" (Red. Szafran M., Kozioł J., Małecka M.), Poznań, , 382-385.

[110] Rickman, Pieper. J., & Barrett, D. M. (2009). Effects of organic and conventional production systems on quality and nutritional parameters of processing tomatoes. J Sci Food Agric, , 89, 177-194.

[111] Rutkowska, G. (1999). Badania zawartości azotanów i azotynów w warzywach uprawianych ekologicznie i konwencjonalnie. Przem. Spoż. , 6, 47-49.

[112] Samaras, J. (1978). Nachernteverhalten unterschiedlich geduengter Gemusearten mit besonderer Berucksichtigung physiologischer und mikrobiologiscer Parameter. Schriftenreihe "Lebendige Erde" Darmstadt.

[113] Schuphan, W. (1974). Nutritional value of crops as influenced by organic and inorganic fertilizer treatments- Qualitas Plantarum- Pl.Fds.hum.Nutr.XIII, , 4, 333-358.

[114] Spadaro, D., Ciavorella, A., Frati, S., Garibaldi, A., & Gullino, M. L. (2008). Occurrence and level of patulin contamination in conventional and organic apple juices marketed in Italy. Poster na konferencji: Cultivating the Future Based on Science: 2nd Conference of the International Society of Organic Agriculture Research ISOFAR, Modena, Italy, June , 18-20.

[115] Stracke, B. A., Rüfer, C. E., Bub, A., Briviba, K., Seifert, S., Kunz, C., & Watzl, B. (2008). Bioavailability and nutritional effects of carotenoids from organically and conventionally produced carrots in healthy men, Br. J. Nutr. Forthcoming, , 1-9.

[116] Sundrum, A., & Acosta, A. Y. (2003). Nutritional strategies to improve the sensory quality and food safety of pork while improving production efficiency within organ-

ic framework conditions. Report of EU-project, Improving Quality and Safety and Reduction of Costs in the European Organic and 'Low Input' Supply Chain, CT-2003 506358.

[117] Szente, V., Szakaly, S., Bukovics, Z. S., Szigeti, O., Polereczki, Z. S., Szekely, O., Berke, S. Z., Takacs, G. Y., Nagyne, Farkas. R., & Szakaly, Z. (2006). The role of CLA content of organic milk in consumers' healthcare. Materiały konferencyjne Joint Organic Congress, Odense, Denmark (www.orgprints.org/7207/).

[118] Szponar, L., & Kierzkowska, E. (1990). Azotany i azotyny w środowisku oraz ich wpływ na zdrowie człowieka. Post.Hig. Med. Dośw. , 44, 327-350.

[119] Tarozzi, A., Hrelia, S., Angeloni, C., Morroni, F., Biagi, P., Guardigli, M., Cantelli-Forti, G., & Hrelia, P. (2006). Antioxidant effectiveness of organically and non-organically grown red oranges in cell culture systems. Eur J Nutr, 45, 152-158.

[120] Taylor, G. C., & Zahradka, P. (2004). Dietary conjugated linoleic acid and insulin sensitivity and resistance in rodent models. American Journal of Clinical Nutrition 79 (Supl.6), 1164S-1168S.

[121] Toledo, P., Andren, A., & Bjorck, L. (2002). Composition of raw milk from sustainable production systems. International Dairy Journal , 12, 75-80.

[122] Toor, R. K., Savage, G. P., & Heeb, A. (2006). Influence of different types of fertilizers on the major antioxidant components of tomatoes. J Food Comp Anal, , 19, 20-27.

[123] Tyburski, J., & Żakowska-Biemans, S. (2007). Wprowadzenie do rolnictwa ekologicznego. Wydawnictwo Szkoły Głównej Gospodarstwa Wiejskiego, Warszawa.

[124] Velimirov, A. (2001). Ratten bevorzugen Biofutter. Oekologie & Landbau , 117, 19-21.

[125] Velimirov, A. (2002). Integrative Qualitaetsmethoden im Zusammenhang mit der P-Wert Bestimmung. Tagungsband 9. Internationale Tagung Elektrochemischer Qualitaetstest, 30.05.-01.06.2002, Institut fuer Gemuesebau und Blumenproduktion, Mendel-Universitaet.

[126] Velimirov, A. (2005). The consistently superior quality of carrots from one organic farm in Austria compared with conventional farms. 15th IFOAM Organic World Congress "Researching and Shaping Sustainable Systems", Adelaide, 21.-23.

[127] Versari, A., Parpinello, G. P., & Mattioli, A. U. (2007). Survey of Patulin Contamination in Italian Apple Juices from Organic and Conventional Agriculture. J of Food Technology, , 5(2), 143-146.

[128] Vogtmann, H. (1985). Ökologischer Landbau- Landwirtschaft mit Zukunft. Pro Natur Verlag, Stuttgart.

[129] Vogtmann, H. (1991). W: Lassen J. Paper- Food Quality and the Consumers. 1993.

[130] Vogtmann, H., Temperli, A. T., Kunsch, U., Eichenberger, M., & Ott, P. (1984). Accumulation of nitrates in leafy vegetables grown under contrasting agricultural systems. Biol Agric Hort, 2, 51 68.

[131] Walshe, B. E., Sheehan, E. M., Delahunty, C. M., Morrissey, P. A., & Kerry, J. P. (2006). Composition, sensory and shelf life stability analyses of Longissimus dorsi muscle from steers reared under organic and conventional production systems. Meat Science , 73, 319-325.

[132] Warman, P. R., & Havard, K. A. (1997). Yield, vitamin and mineral contents of organically and conventionally grown carrots and cabbage. Agriculture, Ecosystems and Environment, , 61, 155-162.

[133] Wawrzyniak, A., Hamułka, J., & Gołębiewska, M. (2004). Ocena zawartości azotanów (V) i azotanów (III) w wybranych warzywach uprawianych konwencjonalnie i ekologicznie. Bromatologia i Chemia Toksykologiczna, , 4, 341-345.

[134] Weibel, F. P., Bickel, R., Leuthold, S., & Alfoldi, T. (2000). Are organically grown apples tastier and healthier? A comparative field study Rusing conventional and alternative methods to measure fruit quality. Acta. Hortic., , 7, 417-427.

[135] Weibel, F. P., Treutter, D., Haseli, A., & Graf, U. (2004). Sensory and health related quality of organic apples: a comparative field study over Tyree years using conventional and holistic methods to assess fruit quality. 11th International Conference on Cultivation Technique and Phyotpathological Problems in Organic Fruit Growing; LVWO: Weinsberg, Germany, , 185-195.

[136] Whigham, L. D., Cook, M. E., & Atkinson, R. L. (2000). Conjugated linoleic acid: implications for human health. Pharmacological Research 42(6), 503-10.

[137] Wieczyńska, J. (2010). rodowiskowe uwarunkowania występowania mikotoksyn w pszenicy ekologicznej i konwencjonalnej. SGGW, Warszawa.

[138] Wilkins, J. L., & Gussow, J. D. (1997). Regional Dietary Guidance: Is the Northeast Nutritionally Complete? Agricultural Production and Nutrition. Proceedings of an International Conference, Boston, Massachusetts, Tufts University, Medford, MA 02155, March 19-21, 1997: 23-33.

[139] Woodward, B. W., & Fernandez, M. I. (1999). Comparison of conventional and organic beef production systems II. Carcass characteristics. Livestock Prod. Sci. , 61, 225-231.

[140] Worthington, V. (2001). Nutritional Quality of Organic Versus Conventional Fruits, Vegetables, and Grains, The Journal of Alternative and Complementary Medicine, 7(2)

[141] Young, J. E., Zhao, X., Carey, E. E., Welti, R., Yang-S, S., & Wang, W. (2005). Phytochemical phenolics in organically grown vegetables. Mol. Nutr. Food Res. , 49, 1136-1142.

[142] Zadoks, J. C. (1989). Development of Farming Systems, Pudoc, Wageningen.

Chapter 5

"Healthy Food" from Healthy Cows

Albert Sundrum

Additional information is available at the end of the chapter

http://dx.doi.org/10.5772/53150

1. Introduction

Milk and milk products are the outcome at the end of a long process and food chain. Various factors on different scales along production and processing can have beneficial or detrimental impacts on various features of dairy products' and process qualities. Indeed, the processes are very complex and far more complex, peculiar and heterogeneous than generally imagined and expected by consumers. On the other hand, the white color of milk and their products provides like a screen an ideal area to project very different attributes and link very different associations with the product while only few reference points are given to validate any of these assumptions.

"Health" implicates a strong attraction for human beings, and food that promises to support and improve health conditions is highly appreciated by consumers. In recent years, consumers' attention to health and food safety issues has increased overwhelmingly because of their increased concern about their own health and the crises and emergencies reported worldwide [1]. "Healthy food from healthy animals" is a slogan often used in the communication between different stakeholders to associate a relationship between the production process, the health status of farm animals and the possible impacts of products from these animals on human health via the consumed food. Although the link is very weak from a scientific point of view (low level of correlation), the associations are strong in the mind of humans and stakeholder groups and effective, especially for the purpose of product marketing.

In the forthcoming sections it is the intention to contribute some enlightenment in the complex process of dairy milk production with a special emphasis on organic production. Without striving for a comprehensive disquisition of the extensive issue, the focus is directed to the question of how expectations of consumers with respect to "healthy food" and the deliveries of organic dairy farmers might fit together. Moreover, which measures might be adequate to bridge the gap between the expectations of different stakeholders involved and what might exceed their potentials? Finally, overall conclusions are drawn with respect to the challenges for organic farmers and for a market driven label program such as organic dairy farming.

2. Expectations of consumers

Consumers are becoming increasingly sensitive about health and welfare problems in commercial livestock production systems, an industry currently under scrutiny for inconsistent practices. More and more consumers expect their food to be produced with greater respect for the needs of farm animals. They express concern about possible hormone, antibiotic, pesticide or chemical residues in animal products and assume that organic products are superior to those produced conventionally in being lower in residues and higher in nutrient content. This largely explains the attention given to this issue as a specific object for public policy and market intervention.

Many consumers also associate organic farming directly with enhanced animal welfare and conflate organic and animal-friendly products [2,3]. For many people, organic farming appears to be a superior alternative to conventional livestock production [4,5]. Consumers' interests and expectations are linked to their willingness to pay premium prices on products which they feel are healthier and safer for their families [6]. In contrast, consumers are less strongly motivated by the altruistic concerns of animal welfare, environmental protection, and the support for rural society – the so-called »public goods«.

Even though organic farming only covers a small percentage of the food market, the expressed sympathy in the general public appears far greater than the market share. Interest in organic food has grown remarkably as consumers react to popular media about health effects and then have gradually evolved attitudes toward the origins and to the production process of food. For example, a change from confinement to grazing systems is one of the tools to evoke positive associations with the product. In this way, animal health and welfare have been turned into quality attributes of food.

Not only the word "health" but also the word "organic" means many different things to consumers. Correspondingly, consumers of organic foods are neither homogenous in demographics nor in beliefs [5,7,8,]. They hold a huge variety of motivations, perceptions, and attitudes regarding organic foods and their consumption. For example, some organic milk consumers buy organic to avoid antibiotics and hormones whereas others focus on different concentrations in valuable ingredients or on the health status of the farm animals. All of these factors drive the decision-making process to buy those products [2].

In contrast to the metaphors and the associated pattern of thought used in sales promotion, consumers' awareness of "healthy food" encounters very complex phenomena, including a large number of factors that have to be taken into account and which are heterogeneous in the outcome. Many consumers do not understand the complexities of organic farming practice and food quality attributes [4]. There is reason to assume that consumers delegate responsibility for ethical issues in food production to the retailer or the government as many consumers do not like to be reminded about issues connected with the animal when choosing products of animal origin [9]. On the other hand, consumer groups mistrust the limited information available at the point of purchase, whereas price is an extremely visible attribute of products related to quality by the notion of value [10]. Demand tends to depend more on the price differential with respect to conventionally grown products than on actual price. In contrast to sensitivity of demand to changes in price, income elasticity of demand for organic foods is generally small [8].

3. Organic agriculture – Based on minimum standards

The International Federation of Organic Agriculture Movements [11] states that organic husbandry focuses on improving animal health and preventing disease through a holistic approach, while at the same time minimizing the use of synthetic medicine. Introduction of the wholesomeness concept in livestock production by organic production is mainly due to a wish for reestablishing a positive image of food safety and animal welfare aspects [12]. Largely, the widespread sympathy for organic agriculture seems to stem from its value-based approach.

Guidelines have been a characteristic feature of organic farming since 1954 when clear criteria have been required by trademark legislation to identify organically produced goods [13]. Because the variety of production sites and the resulting product properties did not allow their identification to be linked to products qualitatively in terms that could be described exactly and understood analytically, the production method itself became the identifying criterion. This fundamental principle has been kept to the present day in the standards of international and national organic agriculture movements and in legislation.

The organic concept refers to the whole farm as the base of a comprehensive system where the production process is intended to ensure quality production rather than maximizing production. The leading idea is based on the voluntary self-restriction in the use of specific means of production with the objectives to produce food of high quality in an animal-appropriate and environment-friendly manner on the basis of a nearly complete nutrient cycle [14]. Organic farming commits itself to a number of substantial values, and thereby sets itself apart from conventional farming. The IFOAM states four principles: (1) Health, (2) Ecology, (3) Fairness, and (4) Care. These principles grew out of stakeholder consultations and were agreed upon on a worldwide basis by the members of IFOAM with each principle being accompanied by an explanation [11]. Nevertheless, organic agriculture is not organized uniformly, neither with respect to the various objectives, nor in the degree of their implementation. There have been and still are different perspectives on organic agriculture with different understandings of what it is and what it develops [15]. A comprehensive definition of organic production is provided by the *Codex Alimentarius* Commission [16].

In Europe, the EU-Regulation (EEC-No. 1804/1999) on organic livestock production, now replaced by EEC-No. 834/2007 was introduced to protect consumers from unjustified claims, to avoid unfair competition between those who label their products as organic, and to ensure equal conditions for all operators. The EU-Regulation provides a framework ensuring living conditions for organic livestock to be better than those in conventional systems, to harmonize the rules across member states, and to make all organic systems subject to minimum standards. Labeling food as being "organic" identifies products as deriving from a production method. In the case of organic products of animal origin minimum standards are defined by specifications for the conversion process, housing conditions, animal nutrition, care and breeding, disease prevention, and veterinary treatment.

According to the EU Regulation, animal health problems shall be controlled mainly by prevention, based on the selection of appropriate breeds or strains of animals, as well as application of animal husbandry practices appropriate to the requirements of each species, and encouraging strong resistance to disease and the prevention of infections. The use of high-quality feed, together with regular exercise and access to pasture, is expected to encourage the natural immunological defense of the animal. Furthermore, an appropriate density of livestock should be ensured, thus avoiding overstocking and any resulting animal health problems.

Concerning veterinary treatment, phytotherapeutic essences and homeopathic products shall be used in preference to chemically synthesized allopathic medicinal products or antibiotics. Where dairy cows receive more than three courses of treatment with chemically synthesized allopathic medicinal products or antibiotics within one year, the livestock concerned, or produce derived from them, may not be sold as being of organic origin. On the other hand, organic farmers are obliged to intervene and treat animals immediately at first signs of illness. In general, the majority of antimicrobial drugs in organic dairy production are used for udder treatments [17,18]. However, due to a lack of control measures, little is known so far as to which degree organic farmers follow the leading ideas of the EU Regulation consistently.

At the international level, the regulation on animal health issue is widely harmonized [19]. Only the US National Organic Program Regulation (NOP) deviates substantially: animal products cannot be sold as certified organic if antibiotics or other substances not listed in the US NOP positive list such as bovine growth hormone, which is used among conventional dairy farmers in the USA to increase milk production, have been used just once. While the US concept seems to be more consumer driven ("pure" food), the European approach considers not only the health aspects of the food but also animal welfare as an important issue.

4. Outcome of minimum standards

As all organic farms are obliged to follow the same minimum standards, one might expect a high level of uniformity in the framework of livestock production and living conditions in comparison to conventional production. However, living conditions for farm animals differ markedly between organic production systems within and between countries [20]. They range from outdoor to indoor production with varying options with respect to space allowance, stocking densities, performance levels, nutrient availabilities, hygiene and air conditions, etc., depending on the farm-specific and local conditions [21]. Although most organic farmers make use of conventional breeds and genotypes, a large variation in the performance level and in the nutrient resources used is found. While feeding rations should be based in the first place on home-grown feedstuffs, they provide a higher variability in ingredients and composition than is expected in the case of feed from the feed mills [22].

In contrast, intensive systems have closely controlled environments to maximize aspects of animal productivity. The equipment of indoor housing and the feeding ration is offered by specialized enterprises, becoming more and more standardized all over the world. Living conditions have typically been adopted across regions and countries, thereby increasing environmental homogeneity between farms and leading to the predominance of a small number of breeds and genotypes that are particularly productive under these specific conditions. Parallel to the increasing performance level, nutrient demands have increased the call for the use of highly concentrated concentrate to meet the nutrient requirements of the animals at their various life stages.

While conventional livestock production has a strong shift toward specialization, the basic concept of organic farming is focused on mixed farms, although the degree of mixture can vary widely [23]. It can be supposed that farmers on highly specialized livestock farms have a more specific management qualification and are more aware of the relevant health-related factors than farmers on mixed farms. Because time capacity and competence of the farmers can be limited, excessive demands in several fields at the same time provoke conflicts within the farm management. In consequence this can lead to deficits on one or more of the various agricultural fields. Thus, there are reasons for the assumption that on organic mixed farms, handling and management of the farm animals are in far greater competition with various other farm activities compared to highly specialized conventional livestock farms.

Thus, the leading ideas and guidelines of organic livestock farming exist only on a meta-level, whereas the implementation in farm practice results in a large variation of living conditions for the farm animals. The complex interactions between different availabilities of resources (labor time, investments, know-how, etc.), different objectives and different priorities thus provide divergent implications on the level of animal health status.

5. Farm animals challenged by multi-factorial diseases

Mastitis, fertility problems, lameness, and metabolic disorders represent the main production diseases within dairy farming throughout the world [24]. These are multi-factorial man-made diseases. They emerge from interactions and synergetic effects between different risk factors and processes which in themselves would not necessarily cause clinical signs of a disease. Their occurrence indicates an overstrained capacity of the farm animals to cope with the living conditions provided by the farm management. To cope with multi-factorial diseases it is of high importance to consider the farm specific conditions, the dynamics and interactions between the various elements of the system, the availability of resources and the ongoing outcome of the interactions. In this respect, animal health status of the herd can be defined as an emergent property of the individual farm system [21].

Thus, the issue of animal health is not primarily related to minimum standards. It largely depends on the capability of the farm management to think through the complexity of the processes on different process levels and to organize a well-balanced farm system and good living conditions for farm animals while facing severe limitations in the availability of relevant resources (labor time, investments, knowledge, etc.). However, living conditions found in practice are so many and diverse that it is often difficult to identify those factors that are most influential and relevant in any actual combination of factors. The challenge to grasp the complexity within a farm system is also hampered by an on-going fragmentation of veterinary and agricultural science into a large number of sub-disciplines with an increasing risk of misinterpretation and misunderstanding [25]. Considerations of single or very few aspects include the risk to oversimplify the matter and to jump to premature conclusions. Relationships between single factors found in experimental studies under *ceteris paribus* assumptions are not always confirmed in epidemiological studies and vice versa, and often do not represent the interactive structure in the farm specific system and situation. Differences between experimental and on-farm conditions shed some doubt on the general applicability of experimental findings for practice.

There is a growing understanding within the scientific community that it is necessary to develop more comprehensive concepts in agricultural science which simultaneously consider a larger number of causal relationships. The isolated view under *ceteris paribus* assumptions is required to be replaced by a systemic approach [26].

6. Milk quality and "healthy milk products"

The term »quality« is documented very diversely in general language use and in the scientific literature. Whilst some understand something very sound and »normal« by this term, others see it rather as something special and extraordinary. According to Mair-Waldburg [27] quality includes both exemptions from deficiencies (inadequacies) as well as the fulfillment of previously determined features (properties) which exceed the usual. For a consumer-orientated quality product it is significant that quality products include a high degree of fulfillment of the consumer's expectation as far as the desired properties are concerned.

Next to the characteristics of the product quality which encompass aspects of nutritional value and hygienic-toxicological, technological and sensory characteristics, consumer expectations also include those related to the production process - so-called »process quality«. According to survey results, many consumers expect that milk originates from healthy animals, produced under animal-friendly husbandry conditions [28].

For some time now, great importance has been ascribed to the content of unsaturated fatty acids, especially the Ω3-fatty acids in milk. Their content in milk is used from various sides in a promotionally effective way to be able to offer consumers a "healthier" milk. In human nutrition the various trans-isomeric fatty acids experience a diverse nutritional evaluation [29]. Whilst trans-fatty acids are assessed negatively, conjugated linoleic acids (CLA) are hoped for. Diverse survey results moreover attribute the Ω3-fatty acids health-promoting effects [30,31]. However according to a meta-analysis, correlating results have not been clearly proven [32].

Research presented by Nielsen & Lund-Nielsen [33] showed organic milk to have higher levels of vitamin E, Ω3-fatty acids, and antioxidant levels than conventional milk. The study concluded that the increased nutritional benefits were due to the organic cows being allowed to graze freely on grass as opposed to being kept in holdings, pens or feed lots. A three-year study in the United Kingdom found organic milk contained 68 percent more Ω3-fatty acids on average than conventional milk [34].

Composition and texture of the milk (especially the protein and fatty acids' content) are very much influenced by the nutrient uptake and nutrient composition [35]. Feeding clover silage, particularly red clover, increases the levels of polyunsaturated fatty acids [36]. A three-fold increase in milk alpha-linolenic acid levels was observed between cows offered red clover silage compared with grass silage. With cows fed with alfalfa and red clover silage, a significant reduction was observed in palmitic acid content of milk. Seasonal effects on the content of fatty acids in milk are primarily due to a modified feed supply. Distinct effects originate from pasture grazing or the intake of greenery compared to feed rations during the winter period [37].

To investigate the effect of the dietary intake of the cow on milk composition, bulk-tank milk was collected on 5 occasions from conventional (n = 15) and organic (n = 10) farms in Denmark and on 4 occasions from low-input nonorganic farms in the United Kingdom, along with management and production parameters [38]. The main results are illustrated in figure 1. The concentration of α-linolenic acid (ALA) was the response variable (Y-variable; the measured output variable that describes the outcome of the experiment), and the amounts of the 8 feed variables were predictors for the organic and conventional milk production systems (X-variables; figure 1A). The regression coefficients (the numerical coefficients that express the link between variation in predictors and variation in response) were significant for the proportion of cereals, pasture, and grass silage in the feed, indicating that these feed components increase the concentration of ALA in milk from the organic and conventional milk production systems. The proportion of maize silage, other silages, by-products, and commercial concentrate mix in the feed gave in contrast a lower ALA concentration in the organic and conventional milk. Moreover, the concentration of linoleic acid (LA) was low in milk from the extensive milk production system, and to identify which feed components in the organic and conventional milk production systems, which had an effect on the concentration of LA in milk, a partial least squares regression analysis (PLS) analysis was performed with the concentration of LA in the milk as response variable and the 8 feed variables as predictors (figure 1B). In this case, the regression coefficients were only significant for the proportion of commercial concentrate mix in the diet, indicating that use of commercial concentrate mix increases the content of LA in organic and conventional milk. However, the proportion of grass silage and other silages in the feed resulted in a low concentration of LA in the milk from the 2 production systems.

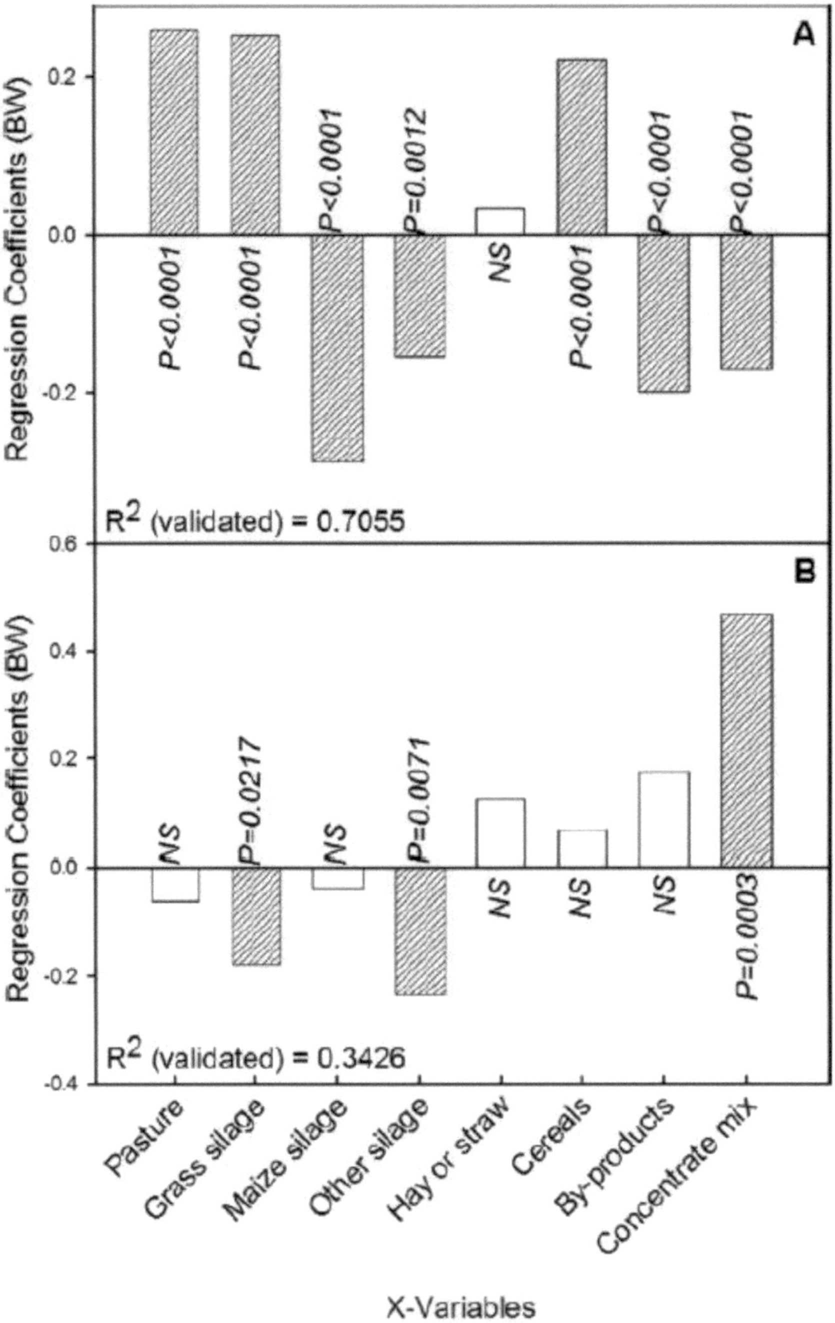

Figure 1. Regression coefficients obtained by partial least squares regression analysis for A) the concentration of α-linolenic acid (C18:3n-3) in organic and conventional milk and B) the concentration of linoleic acid (C18:2n-6) in organic and conventional milk as response variable with the feed variables as predictors (X-variables) minus the vitamin supplement. The bars with diagonal stripes are significant; NS = non-significant (Slots et al., 2009).

According to the results found in trials in mountainous regions, milk from cows which only fed from greenery from alpine pastures showed a higher content Ω3-fatty acid than a comparable group of cows with silage feed [39]. The nutritional content of grass greenery is decisive for the fatty acid profile of the total milk fat regardless of the altitude of the pasture region [40]. The positive effect of silage feed and/or pasture feeding on the composition of fatty acid can be associated with a lower lacto-protein (41,42]. However, an increased Ω3-fatty acid content is not linked only to pasture grazing. Additives of vegetable fats, e.g. linseed oil, provoke similar effects as pasture grazing [43].

Although grazing in general provides a positive effect on the content of fatty acids in milk, buying organic milk does, unfortunately, not guarantee that one is buying milk from open pasture grass-grazing cows. Instead of pasture grazing, organic farmers in Europe are allowed to offer an outdoor area without any grass available. Moreover, access to pasture and feed quality of clover-grass is restricted and depending on the vegetation period, widely varying between regions and farms as does the daily time period cows are enabled or not able to spend on pasture.

Unfortunately, there are further constraints that act against the general trend of simplifying mental associations between grazing and "healthy milk". In the accessible literature there is reference that the contents of free fatty acids including the Ω3-fatty acids increase in connection with the inflammatory reaction in the udder [44]. A further survey brought to light that free fatty acids in the milk of clinically infected areas of the udder were in a six times higher concentration than in the non-infected udder area of the same cows [45]. Should these relationships be confirmed in further studies, an increased content of Ω3-fatty acids in the milk cannot be judged unreservedly positive, but only in connection with the status of udder health.

Mastitis does not only include a high content of Ω3-fatty acids in the milk but goes along with numerous impacts on milk quality: high somatic cell counts, high levels of bacteria in milk, high amounts of antibiotics used with the risk of antibiotic residue failures and the development of antimicrobial resistance, clinical signs with pain, suffering and tissue damage for the dairy cows.

Udder diseases are associated with minor up to high degree damage of the mammary tissue [46]. Often chronic progression of the disease and thereby irreversible modifications in the glandular tissue takes place. Furthermore, the animals suffer more or less distinct pain perception and general discomfort [47,48]. Functionality of other body organs can also be considerably affected [49]. High rates of illness in the herd with limited therapeutic success determine an increased culling rate [50,51]. After fertility disorders, udder diseases portray the second most frequent causes for culling of dairy cows from the herd [52].

Local and systemic reactions of the organism on penetrated foreign germs alter the content of immune defense cells and antibodies as well as the content of electrolytes and trace elements [53]. Subject to the degree of severity, the inflammation processes in the udder tissue always go hand in hand with losses in quality of the milk for human consumption. An increased cell and salinity [54], a reduction of the casein content, an increase of the pH-value, a reduction of the cheese dairy efficiency and clearly increased lipolysis and proteolysis activity contribute to this [55]. The increased enzyme activity does not only impair the sensoric properties of milk, but also negatively affects the shelf-life of pasteurized and refrigerated storage of milk [56] as well as the cheese yield and storage [57,58].

The udder health status of dairy cows portrays a fundamental criterion of animal health. From the veterinarian perspective, an udder area (quarter) is then seen as healthy if the content of somatic cells in the milk does not exceed the figure of 100,000 cells/ml milk and with a bacteriologic test of the milk that there are no pathogens proven [59,60]. In contrast, the EU-Regulation (EC-No 853/2004) for bulk tank milk fixes the marginal value of 400,000 cells/ml in the geometric mean from three months for tradable milk. In the USA, the current legal limit for bulk tank SCC is even higher and fixed on 750,000 cells/ml for Grade A producers [61]. On the other hand, the EU-Regulation demands that raw milk must be from animals which are free of any signs of an infection which can be transmitted to humans via the milk. They must have good health and may not be suffering from a visible udder inflammation and udder wounds, which could affect the milk disadvantageously. While the inconsistencies within the EU Regulation are obvious, the utilization of milk from cows which suffer from subclinical mastitis is not explicitly prohibited by legislation. The threshold values with respect to milk quality ordinance bear no relation to udder health.

Nevertheless, in practice BTSCC levels beyond the legal marginal value are often associated with a tolerable udder health status. Although the concentration of germs and somatic cells in the milk deriving from dairy farms is generally high, this does not comprehend a problem for the issue of food safety as the milk is pasteurized. The exclusion of health risks for the consumers to a large extent might be the main reason why consumers and retailers are largely inert against the health and welfare problems in dairy herds.

Summing up, although defined by basic guidelines, organic livestock production is characterized by largely heterogeneous farming conditions that allow for huge differences in the availability of nutrient resources, housing conditions, genotypes and management skills, all of which variously impact milk quality and animal health. Correspondingly, there is substantial variation in the product and process quality of organic milk already within each herd. The milk of heterogeneous quality from different farms is delivered to the dairy, mixed to a homogeneous raw product with defined raw ingredients (especially fat content), while any top quality is down and worse quality is upgraded before the milk enters the market.

7. Status of animal health in organic dairy production

Several scientifically based studies on how and to what degree the EU-Regulation contributes to the objective of a high status of animal health in organic farming have been conducted in the last decade [62,63]. Still many open questions remain, especially with respect to the implementation of the gained scientific knowledge into practice. The assessment of animal health is a difficult task facing a high level of complexity due to the various interactions between health influencing factors. In the literature, huge differences and inter-country variation exist in study designs and quality of the studies. Complexity arises with current definitions of disease that includes subclinical conditions and a health management that considers animal health as herd performance [64]. Difficulties with methodology are also related to the health indicators in use. Indeed, good records are available only for the most easily diagnosed diseases. In this context, there is a need for a critical assessment of routinely collected health-related data used in research in order to make valid inferences regarding animal health performance [65].

Mastitis causes substantial economic losses and hampers animal welfare for both organic and conventional farmers. Differing results have been reported for udder health when organic and conventional dairy herds were compared. Based on treatment data from the Norwegian Cattle Health Service, no significant differences in the mean values of somatic cell counts (SCC) were found [66]. In a Swedish study, organic dairy cows tend to have higher somatic cell counts than non-organic cows [67]. In contrast, Garmo *et al.* [68] found that organic cows had lower milk SCC and a lower mastitis treatment rate than conventional cows. In Denmark, in a study involving 27 organic and 57 conventional herds, the percentage of cows treated for mastitis per month was 1.8–5.1 (25% and 75% percentiles) in organic herds and 3.3–6.7 in conventional herds [69]. Other studies show varying results including better udder health on organic farms [70], no difference [71] and higher levels of mastitis on organic farms [72].

Surveys from Switzerland, Norway, Sweden, Germany and the UK suggest that organic dairy herds do not have more fertility related problems than conventional herds [62]. In contrast, the calving interval and the intervals from calving to first and last artificial insemination (AI) were shorter for organic compared to conventional cows [73]; or showed only marginal differences between organic and conventional farms in reproductive performance [74]. An impaired reproductive performance in organic cows has been reported from Norway [75]. The differences from conventional production were due to a limited energy intake and longer winter season in the organic cows.

So far only a few investigations have been conducted to assess lameness in organic herds. Lameness plays a considerable role in organic dairy farming as demonstrated in a pilot study in 50 organic dairy herds in Germany [76]. Lower levels of lameness in organic farms than in non-organic units were found in a study by Rutherford *et al.* [77]. With the purpose of explaining the variance of different claw disorders, Holzhauer *et al.* [78] emphasized that herd-level factors are most important for the prevalence of hoof lesions.

The context of milk productivity may play a pivotal role in adaptation in the pathogenesis of metabolic disorders in relation to negative energy balance, such as excessive lipid accumulation in the liver, ketosis, abomasal displacement, cystic ovarian disease and laminitis [79]. In fact, surveys report lower production levels in the organic managed herds and support a yield-based explanation of any differences in metabolic or digestive disorder levels [62]. The incidence of clinical ketosis reported in most comparative studies was similar or even lower in organic than in conventional herds [80]. In the Swedish context, Fall *et al.* [71] and Blanco-Penedo *et al.* [81] found no significant differences in clinical ketosis between organic and conventional herds, which included the change of legislation towards 100% organic diet. Regarding micro-mineral status, it has been suggested that selenium status may be poorer in organic compared to conventional farms [82].

Accounting for other health indicators, longevity is a reflection of the cow's ability to avoid being culled. In Norway, cows in organic husbandry live longer [75] whereas results of a study in Sweden showed only marginal differences between organic and conventional farms in the length of productive life [74]. The rate of culling due to mastitis in Sweden was found to be similar in 26 organic herds and 1102 conventional herds [70]. In a recent study of Swedish organic herds, the overall most common reason for culling was poor udder health followed by low fertility and leg problems [83]. The ranking order in culling reasons differed in comparison to conventional herds. Studies that have compared health performance in conventional and organic farms have shown that disease problems in organic milk production tend to be similar (metabolic problems, lameness and mastitis in dairy cows) to what is found under conventional conditions while the extent of these problems varies considerably among farms [84], and between European countries [63].

Currently, a considerable number of organic farms cannot cope, in all respects, with the requests for high animal health status. As differences between farms appear to be greater than those between production methods, organic livestock farming defined by minimum standards does not provide a homogenous outcome with respect to animal health [85]. Obviously, the issue of animal health often is not the first priority in organic livestock farming.

Striving for a high status of animal health requires high management skills; one must be capable to gain an overall picture of the complex interactions within a farming system, to reflect on the most relevant factors, to implement feedback mechanisms, and guide the production process. Thus, it primarily depends on the management as to whether the potentials for a high level of animal health are fully realized. Differences in management practices, restrictions in the availability of resources (such as labor time, financial budget), and a lack of feedback and control mechanism within the farm system appear to be primary reasons for the substantial variation.

8. What prevents organic farmers from improving animal health status?

Reasons for the current unsatisfactory situation in organic dairy farming are manifold and differ considerably between farms as do the prevalence rates of multi-factorial production diseases. Identifying the main causes for the specific problems as well as the main constraints in farm management practices is essential when striving for improvements in animal health. Thus, a profound diagnostic procedure at different scales (animal, herd, and farm level) is the starting point of any initiatives.

Previous herd health planning has contributed to improving farm management and has prepared the ground for further advancements [63]. However, recommended measures have often been implemented in the daily farm practice only to a low degree. Thus, weak success

http://dx.doi.org/10.5772/53150

has been achieved so far by traditional herd health planning and management, differing widely between farms. To reduce the prevalence of multi-factorial diseases it is required in the first place to identify and remove the main causes and risk factors of diseases therewith taking into account the whole farm context. On many farms the bottle neck for any improvements might be due to limitations in the ability to think through the complexity of the production processes on the different scales. Many farmers are trapped in their own perspective and are often left alone when assessing, diagnosing and treating farm animals without a valid reference point and without any control by a veterinarian authority or certification bodies whether they are successful or not in their efforts to improve the animal health status.

Because time capacities are limited, excessive demands in several fields at the same time provoke conflicts, leading to deficits in one or more of the agricultural fields. The need for additional labor efforts and increasing cost for health improvements often are constraints that prevent farmers from seeking advice and making use of recommended measures. In this context, it is often argued that farmers will benefit from a high status of animal health by higher performance and lower veterinary costs and thus should have an inherent incentive to reduce the occurrence of diseases. This conclusion seems comprehensible as production diseases have a serious impact on the productivity of a dairy farm by reducing the efficiency with which resources (e.g. feedstuffs) are converted into products [86].

However, from a different perspective, this widespread pattern of thought, frequently observed in different stakeholder groups including veterinary and agricultural science, belongs to a severe error in reasoning. It leaves the responsibility by the farmer for not being clever enough to make use of a high level of animal health as a relevant source of a higher income by reducing the production costs. This approach declares all farmers facing a high prevalence rate of production diseases, at least indirectly, as being stupid, an accusation which would - on the base on the prevalence rates mentioned above – apply to the majority of dairy farmers. In contrast, our own studies give reason to the conclusion that farmers might react quite reasonably as economic calculations on a high number of dairy farms in Germany showed that a high animal health status in general does not increase farmers' income [87].

The previous pattern of thought is an example for a restricted perspective, fading out relevant facts, in this case the costs for prevention and control of diseases. Generally, cost factors for dairy production diseases are restricted to those for cow replacements, veterinary services, diagnostics, drugs, discarded milk, labor efforts, decreased performance, decreased milk quality, increased risk of new cases of the same disease or of other diseases [88]. In daily farmers' lives, costs for treatment are often seen as a part of the losses due to the occurrence of disease but not as an additional input to reduce the losses through diseases.

According to Hogeveen [89], it is more practical to talk about failure costs and preventive costs instead of talking losses and expenditures. The higher the preventive costs, the lower the failure costs and vice versa. Because the relation between prevention and failure is not linear, there is an optimal level of control in relation to economic considerations. Because the production functions as well as the failure costs and preventive costs vary considerably from farm to farm, the optimal level of control is farm specific and cannot be generalized. In a Dutch study on 120 conventional dairy farms, costs of prevention in the case of mastitis were made up to more than 75% by costs for labor and were predominantly higher than the total failure costs [90].

The cost and labor intensive efforts for preventive measures and the uncertainties with respect to their effectiveness explain to some degree why farmers are reluctant to increase the efforts for prevention in order to reduce the prevalence rates of diseases and the failure costs deriving therefrom. The success of preventive measures is dependent to a high degree on the expertise and the persuasive power of those who give advice. Without a validation process with respect to the given advice, there is a high risk that the advice fails to be effective and efficient. Correspondingly, cost-benefit calculations of recommended measures are essential to convince the farmer into action. Future research work is needed which focuses on the cost-effectiveness of preventive measures under various farm conditions.

However, profound knowledge alone is not sufficient to change the current unsatisfactory situation. Indeed, no progress can be expected with regard to animal health if farmers do not gain any benefit and profit from the market to compensate for the additional efforts and resources needed to improve farm management and health status. Currently, producers are very much at the mercy of retailers and supermarkets in terms of price paid per liter of milk. These are continuously trying to drop their milk price to producers. As a consequence, dairy farmers have been chronically underpaid in recent years and left alone by the market, which does not offer any monetary incentives to improve the animal health status on the farms.

The current market conditions widely ignore the large variability in quality traits and in the impacts on common goods, promoting unfair competition when enabling equal prices for very different performances in relation to product and process qualities. Farmers who gain economic benefits by selling organic products to premium prices but only providing a low level of animal health undermine the efforts of other farmers attempting to maintain a high level of animal health [91]. In general, the latter have to apply additional labor and cost intensive efforts, contributing to considerably increase their production costs while at the same time providing an essential competitive disadvantage.

9. Animal health as a marketable quality trait

The processes of production, processing and marketing of organic milk occur on different scales, within different systems and involve different stakeholder groups. Concluding, they can be characterized as being quite complex. Each stakeholder group has its own perspective on the scenery, overlooking some but seldom gain an encompassing overview about the main driving forces, potentials or constraints along the food chain. Kahneman [92] deserves the particular merit to have brought the issue of perception and decision making within economic affairs into the focus of a broader public. In the face of the enlightening findings by neurophysiology, cognition science and psychology, the *homo oeconomicus* as a basic model of economic science does more look like a legendary creature than a real person in life. Also other disciplines are challenged to rethink the axioms and assumptions of their disciplines.

http://dx.doi.org/10.5772/53150

According to Kahneman [92], the operations of associative memory contribute to a general confirmation bias. Contrary to the rules of philosophers of science, who advise testing hypotheses by trying to refute them, people (and scientists, quite often) seek data that are likely to be compatible with the beliefs they currently hold. Jumping to conclusions on the bases of limited evidence is a main process of intuitive thinking, being radically insensitive to both the quality and the quantity of information that gives rise to impressions and intuitions. It is the consistency of the information that matters for a good story, not its completeness. Indeed, knowing little makes it easier to fit everything one knows into a coherent pattern. The associative machinery suppresses ambiguity and spontaneously constructs stories that are as coherent as possible. Unless the message is immediately negated, the associations that it evokes will spread as if the message were true. Thus, humans are in the first place pattern seekers, believers in a coherent world, in which regularities appear not by accident but as a result of mechanical causality or of someone's intention. People can maintain an unshakable faith in any position, however absurd, when they are sustained by a community of like-minded believers.

The previous excursion, although only a foretelling of what requires a comprehensive reflection concerning the impacts on agricultural and veterinary sciences, gives a hint why stakeholder groups are striving for coherency in their world view and patterns of thinking within their community and are prone to ignore and fad out all those aspects that might disturb this coherency. From a scientific point of view, there is need to focus especially on the inconsistencies in statements and conclusions within and between the stakeholder groups involved. Some of the various discrepancies between claim and reality with respect to the handling of the animal health issue in organic and conventional livestock production and some of the conflicting areas provoked therewith are described below [21]:

- Retailers and/or producers claim to offer products that derive from healthy animals, without providing transparency and evidence of animal health status of farm animals.
- Retailers want to increase the turnover by offering organic food with comparable low prices and at the expense of the possibilities of the farmer to investigate substantial improvements of animal health.
- Producers who strive for a high status of animal health by using appropriate management concepts and encountering higher production costs are confronted with unfair competition when competing with their products on the same markets as those who produce on a low cost and low quality base.
- A high percentage of consumers announces their special interest in the issue of animal health and their willingness to pay premium prices, but hesitates to do so when corresponding food is offered and instead prefers purchasing cheaper food.
- Many consumers prefer to delegate responsibility for ethical issues when choosing animal products to the retailer or the government and are by their ignorance jointly responsible for the severe deficits in animal health within livestock production.

Possible expectations of consumers that specific food might improve their own health status can be seen as part of a general oversimplification. As described above in relation to animal health, the issue of health is very complex and the aspect of nutrient intake is only one of many risk factors. Thus, it is very difficult to provide evidence for a direct impact of specific food on human health.

In Europe, the Regulation on nutrition and health claims made on foods (EC No 1924/2006) was adopted by the Council and Parliament to prevent misuse. It foresees implementing measures to ensure that any claim made on foods' labeling, presentation or marketing in the European Union is clear, accurate and based on evidence accepted by the whole scientific community. Consequently foods bearing claims that could mislead consumers will be eliminated from the market.

In contrast, it is possible to promote products deriving from healthy animals. However, such an advertising message should also be based on evidence. Due to the complexity of the interactions of various factors on different scales, evidence cannot refer to some input variables, e.g. minimum standards, but have to focus on the outcome of process. The appropriate reference point for the output orientation within a systemic approach is the animal health status of the individual farm. Health is the emergent outcome of the processes within a farm system. The farm system is the functional unit and system of the production process. It is characterized by boundaries and steered by the farm manager who is challenged to balance the potentials and limitations of the production conditions, the available resources and the conflicting areas provoked by limitations. The farm specific animal health status is the result of the steering process and as such the emergent property of the farm system. Within a label program such as organic, quality assurance and control programs for products labeled as deriving from healthy herds and animals can rely on fixed levels concerning the acceptable prevalence rate of diseases.

As the somatic cell count (SCC) from lactating cows are quantified monthly as a routine on nearly all farms, extensive data material is available which can be used for farm internal feedback analysis and improvements and simultaneously as a diagnostic tool with respect to the udder health of the dairy cows in the herd. Thresholds which define an acceptable status of udder health have been described by several authors [93]. For example, those farms which take part in a label program of top quality milk should provide milk with less than 150,000 somatic cell counts in the bulk tank (BTSCC), and the incidence of clinical mastitis (ICM) should not exceed the rate of 0,33 (cases per average cow in the farm per year).

Current data evaluations show that for instance approximately 11% of the Bavarian dairy cows exceed the threshold value of over 400,000 SCC/ml in the bulk tank milk [87]. These counts mark the top of a distinct ‚cell mountain'. In a study on 120 conventional dairy farms, the incidence of clinical mastitis showed a huge variation between 0.03 to 1.21 [90], therewith indicating the need to provide orientation and define a threshold that should not be exceeded. Due to the various impacts of udder diseases on relevant traits of milk quality, including risks due to residues and the development of antibacterial resistance, the recommended thresholds are suited to mark a distinction between different levels of both product and process quality.

Data of both BTSCC and ICM are resp. should be available on organic dairy farms, and hence do not require additional efforts for their assessment. Consequently, the possible occurrence of enormous additional bureaucratic expenditures cited as possible counter-argumentation can be rejected. Nevertheless, the separated obtaining and processing of milk from farms with a high animal health status will definitely increase costs. The main question is what it worth is to produce and consume milk from healthy dairy cows.

The trade value of milk is determined primarily by quantity of milk and milk content while qualitative traits are currently of no relevance and an outstanding quality is not rewarded by higher prices. Without evidence based progress, organic livestock production faces the risk to lose the confidence of the consumers while being trapped between own demands, consumer expectations and limited resources [94]. Thus, there is need for an evidence based system of financial penalties and bonus payments to promote top quality milk. Despite the fact that many consumers express their wish for high quality products, the current payment and marketing systems counteract all efforts to follow consumer demands and fail to communicate adequately differentiated milk quality. Conclusion is that only a direct assessment of animal health and a payment system that honors quality grades beyond average can contribute to improve the currently unsatisfying situation. This, however, requires a shift in the paradigm from a guideline and input oriented to an output oriented approach, and the implementation of a systematic approach for an effective and efficient balancing of the multiple variables and complex interactions within each farming system.

10. Conclusions

Organic farming has committed itself to outperforming conventional farming in a number of areas including animal health. However, organic standards based on minimum requirements do not automatically lead to a high status of animal health that exceeds the level in conventional production and thus, does not in all respects meet consumers' expectations. Improvements are crucial to support and strengthen consumers' confidence and their willingness to pay premium prices. These are urgently needed to cover the higher production costs in organic farming and thus ensure a viable organic dairy production.

According to previous knowledge, assessments of the quality of organic milk provides inconsistent results and often falls short of expectations as it is often similar or even lower than the quality of conventionally produced milk. In view of the large heterogeneity between organic farms in relation to both living conditions of the farm animals and the status of animal health, it appears to have been a congenital failure of organic agriculture to have neglected the definition of minimum standards with respect to the qualitative outcome of the production process, especially the status of animal health.

While farmers as owners are initially responsible for the well-being of their farm animals, they are very limited in their options of decision-making as they, in general, possess little financial flexibility that can be used for improvements. In the past, a clear increase in the productivity of milk production has led to a remarkable decrease of milk prices in relation to the general income from which the consumers have benefited in the first place. While there might have been time periods when the majority of farmers and also farm animals have gained advantage from technical innovations, these times have definitely gone. Dairy cows pay the continuous increase in productivity and milk yield with an increase in the prevalence rates of production diseases and with a decrease in longevity [52]. Farmers are facing a high volatility of milk prices. In recent years, they have gone through a long phase of milk prices which did not cover the total production costs. Correspondingly, the number of dairy farmers who had to quit has increased dramatically. The predominant competition is based on the reduction of prices while widely ignoring the internal and external costs that emerge from these processes. In Europe, the phase-out of the Milk Quota Regulation in 2015 will fuel the competition even more. In face of the shortfall to be financed, the increase in herd size and the decrease in available resources (labor time and investments), there is reason to assume that the situation in the future will become even worse. While the market fails to provide different levels of product and process quality, national governments fail to prevent unfair competition on the market. On the other hand, they are not forced by the majority of voters to initiate and chair changes in the predominating structures of the market.

From the farmers' perspective, to honor a higher health status by premium prices, and to reduce unfair competition are of great importance to improve the unsatisfying situation. The market, however, fails to provide incentives for any quality improvements, often blaming the consumers for not being prepared to pay adequate premium prices. On the other hand, the consumers are not appropriately informed about the current level of product and process quality and are misguided by sales promotion. It is generally accepted in the market economy that the stakeholders being part of the food chain are striving for their own benefit in the first place. In the complex interactions between stakeholders groups, the players generally pose in active as well as in passive roles, and are both victims and offenders. In general, the strength of one actor is based on the weakness of the other stakeholders. While farm animals and farmers are in a very weak position, retailers and supermarkets are in a strong position to beat down the price in order to increase the turnover rates and their profit. Nevertheless, they can only act in such a way because consumer groups are dominated by bargain hunters, and those who are largely ignoring the problems of the other stakeholders, including health and welfare problems of the farm animals. Consumers are able to make a choice between large ranges of products without being able to assess their quality. Expenditures for food in relation to the total budget of a household have dramatically decreased during the last few decades. Hence, consumers in general can afford more expensive food products if their priorities are inclined in this fashion. However, consumers have become used to very low food prices while imagining they are on the safe side concerning the quality issue.

So far estimations of consumers with respect to traits of food and process quality are primarily based on associations and on expectations deriving therefrom. They are definitely not evidence based. Large variations in features that are relevant for those who buy organic products meet with large variations in the factual results of quality traits. Currently, the complexity of processes within the food production chain is reduced primarily to the quantifiable size of the price stakeholders receive or have to pay for the intermediate or the final product. However, prices for intermediate or final dairy products are unreal for their part as they do not represent and include the entity of the internal and external costs of the production process, e.g. the worse ani-

http://dx.doi.org/10.5772/53150

mal health situation for dairy cows, and the non-covering of the productions costs, let alone the environmental impacts due to the high amounts of nutrient losses and emissions of greenhouse gas caused by the processes of production and processing. While consumers could afford higher milk prices, only few and not enough are willing to face the problems, caused by the impacts of their buying behavior and by the unfair competition within the market. As long as not enough producers are willing to enlighten the consumers about the real production conditions and as long as not enough consumers are not really interested to get an inside view into the production processes, the discrepancies between demands and reality of organic and conventional dairy production is expected to continue.

One of the most frequently asked questions in western society: who is to blame for malfunction, does not provoke an easy and obvious answer as all human stakeholders are part of a production system that is based on exploitation of land area, and farm animals, some to a higher and some to a lesser degree. Currently, stakeholder groups involved are not prepared to rethink their dominating pattern of thoughts and are not willing to risk the possible need for changes when having a closer look at the living conditions of farm animals and the impacts on product and process quality. The persisting power is still too high to provide a chance for real improvements. While some stakeholders are trapped in inherent necessities with very small degrees of freedom in decision making, consumers are free to decide on what they spend their money and are benefitting simultaneously from very low food prices. Correspondingly, they could be blamed in the first place for their ignorance towards the impacts of their buying behavior on the production process and on animal health and welfare. Any complaints by consumers with respect to the low level of product and process quality, either in conventional or in organic dairy production, should be rejected.

In general, food does not exert a direct influence on human health but is well known for providing both positive and/or negative impacts on the capability of the organism to cope with the various and specific demands. Thus, the slogan "healthy food from healthy animals" represents an abbreviated mental association, not being scientifically sound. However, the slogan is applicable and valid in the way that only milk from healthy cows with healthy udders is delivering the starting product for milk products of top quality. Currently, milk and milk products which derive exclusively and evidence based from healthy cows are not available on the market. If consumers really want food from healthy cows they have to establish a corresponding demand and have to reject those products that do not fulfill this demand.

Author details

Albert Sundrum*

Address all correspondence to: sundrum@uni-kassel.de

Department of Animal Nutrition and Animal Health, University of Kassel, Witzenhausen, Germany

References

[1] Canavari M., Olson KD. (eds.), Organic food. Consumers' choices and farmers' opportunities. Springer, New York; 2007.

[2] Harper GC., Makatouni A. Consumer perception of organic food production and farm animal welfare. Br. Food J. 2002; 104:287-299.

[3] McEachern MG., Willock J. Producers and consumers of organic meat: A focus on attitudes and motivations. Brit. Food J. 2004; 106:534-552.

[4] Yiridoe E., Bonti-Ankomah S., Martin R. Comparison of consumer perceptions and preferences toward organic versus conventionally-produced foods: a review and update of the literature. Renewable Agriculture and Food Systems 2005; 20, 193–205.

[5] Hughner RS., McDonagh P., Prothero A. Who are organic food consumers? A compilation and review of why people purchase organic food. Journal of Consumer Behaviour 2007; 6:94–110.

[6] Zanoli Z. (ed.) The European Consumer and Organic Food OMiaRD Vol. 4. University of Wales, Aberystwyth (UK), pp175; 2004.

[7] Aertsens J., Verbeke W., Mondelaers K., Van Huylenbroeck G. Personal determinants of organic food consumption: a review. 2009; Br. Food J. 111:1140-1167.

[8] Martelli G. Consumers' perception of farm animal welfare: an Italian and European perspective. Ital. J. Anim. Sci. 2009; 8:31-41.

[9] Skarstad F., Terragni L., Torjusen H. Animal welfare according to Norwegian consumers and producers: definitions and implications. Int. J. Sociology of Food and Agriculture 2007; 15:74–90.

[10] McEachern MG., Schröder MJ. The role of livestock production ethics in consumer values towards meat. J. Agric. Environ. Ethics 2002; 15:221-237.

[11] IFOAM (International Federation of Organic Agricultural Movement) Principles of Organic Agriculture, Bonn, Germany; 2006.

[12] Verbeke W A., Viaene J. Ethical challenges for livestock production: meeting consumer concerns about meat safety and animal welfare. J. Agric. Environ. Ethics. 2000; 12:141-151.

[13] Schaumann W. Der wissenschaftliche und praktische Entwicklungsweg des oekologischen Landbaus und seine Zukunftsperspektive. In: Schaumann W., Siebeneicher G., Luenzer I. (eds) Geschichte des oekologischen Landbaus. SOEL-Sonderausgabe 2002;65:11–58.

[14] Sundrum A. EEC-Regulation on organic livestock production and their contribution to the animal welfare issue, in: KTBL (ed.), Regulation of Animal Production in Europe. KTBL-Schrift 1999; 270:93–97.

[15] Alroe HF., Noel E. What makes organic agriculture move - protest, meaning or market? A polyocular approach to the dynamics and governance of organic agriculture. Int. J. Agric. Res. Governance and Ecology 2008; 7:5–22.

[16] Codex Alimentarius Commission. Guidelines for the production, processing, labelling and marketing of organically produced foods 1999: Amended 2010.

[17] Menéndez González S., Steiner A., Gassner B., Regula G. Antimicrobial use in Swiss dairy farms: Quantification and evaluation of data quality. Preventive Veterinary Medicine 2010; 95:50–63.

[18] Wagenaar JP., Klocke P., Butler G., Smolders G., Nielsen J., Canever A., Leifert C. Effect of production system, alternative treatments and calf rearing system on udder health in organic dairy cows. NJAS - Wageningen Journal of Life Sciences 2011; 58:157–162.

[19] Schmid O., Huber B., Ziegler K., Jespersen LM., Plakolm G. Analysis of differences between EU Regulation 2092/91 in relation to other standards. In: Proc. 16th IFOAM Org. World Congr. "Cultivate the future" and the 2nd Sci. Conf. "Cultivating the future based on science" of ISOFAR (Int. Soc. Org. Agric. Res.). Vol. 2. June 18–20th, p382–385; 2008.

[20] Vaarst M., Padel S., Younie D., Sundrum A., Hovi M., Rymer C. The SAFO project: outcomes, conclusions and challenges for the Future, In: Rymer C., Vaarst M., Padel S. (eds.), Future perspective for animal health on organic farms: main findings, conclusions and recommendations from SAFO Network Proceedings of the 5th SAFO Workshop, Odense, Denmark; 2006.

[21] Sundrum A. Health and welfare of organic livestock and its challenges. In: Ricke SC., Van Loo EJ., Johnson MG., O'Bryan CA. (eds.) Organic meat production and processing. Wiley-Blackwell, p89-112; 2011.

[22] Sundrum A., Nicholas P., Padel S. Organic farming: challenges for farmers and feed suppliers, in: Garnsworthy, P., Wiseman, J. (Eds.), Recent Advances in Animal Nutrition 2007. Nottingham University Press, p239–260; 2008.

[23] Hermansen J., Kristensen T. Research and evaluation of mixed farming systems for ecological animal production in Denmark, In: van Keulen H. (ed.), Mixed farming systems in Europe: workshop proceedings Dronten, The Netherlands, p97–101; 1998.

[24] Rushton J. The economics of animal health and production: A practical and theoretical guide. CABI, Wallingford; 2009.

[25] Zinsstag J., Schelling E., Waltner-Toews D., Tanner M. From "one medicine" to "one health" and systemic approaches to health and well-being. Preventive Veterinary Medicine 2011; 101:148–156.

[26] DFG (German Research Foundation) Future perspectives of agricultural science and research. Wiley-VCH publisher, Bonn, Germany; 2005.

[27] Mair-Waldburg H. Qualitätsmanagement - Qualitätssicherung. In: Handbuch Milch, Kap 3: Qualität und Qualitätssicherung, Hamburg; 2002.

[28] Grunert KG., Beck-Lasen T., Bredahl L. Three issues in consumer quality perception and acceptance of dairy products. Int. Dairy J. 2000; 10:575-584.

[29] Jahreis G., Kraft J., Michel P. Milch vom Nutzerzeugnis zum Designerprodukt. Sonderheft 242, Landbauforschung Völkenrode 2002; p13-23.

[30] Psota TL., Gebauer SK., Kris-Etherton P. Dietary omega-3 fatty acid intake and cardiovascular risk. Am. J. Cardiol. 2006; 98:3i-18i.

[31] Gleissman H., Segerström L., Hamberg M., Ponthan F., Lindskog JI., Kogner P. Omega-3 fatty acid supplementation delays the progression of neuroblastoma in vivo. Int. J. Cancer. 2011; 128 (7) 1703-1711.

[32] Hooper L., Thompson RL., Harrison RA., Summerbell CD., Ness AR., Moore HJ., Worthington HV., Durrington PN., Higgins JP., Capps NE., Riemersma RA., Ebrahim SB., Smith GD. Risks and benefits of omega 3 fats for mortality, cardiovascular disease, and cancer: systematic review. BMJ. 2006; 332:752-760.

[33] Nielsen JH., Lund-Nielsen T. Healthier organic livestock products; antioxidants in organic and conventional produced milk. Book of Abstract. First Annual Congress of the EU Project Quality Low Input Food and the Soil Association Annual Conference. Newcastle, 6-9 January; 2005.

[34] Ellis K., Innocent G., Grove-White D., Cripps P., McLean WG., Howard CV., Mihm M. Comparing the fatty acid composition of organic and conventional milk. J. Dairy Sci. 2006; 89:1938-1950.

[35] Lock AL., Bauman DE. Modifying milk fat composition of dairy cows to enhance fatty acids beneficial to human health. Lipids 2004; 3912:1197-1206.

[36] Dewhurst RJ., Fisher WJ., Tweed JK., Wilkins RJ. Comparison of grass and legume silages for milk production. Production responses with different levels of concentrate. J. Dairy Sci. 2003; 86:2598-2611.

[37] Butler G., Nielsen JH., Slots T., Seal C., Eyre MD., Sanderson R., Leifert C. Fatty acid and fat-soluble antioxidant concentrations in milk from high- and low-input conventional and organic systems: seasonal variation. 2008; J. Sci. Food Agric. 88:1431-1441.

[38] Slots T., Butler G., Leifert C., Kristensen T., Skibsted LH., Nielsen JH. Potentials to differentiate milk composition by different feeding strategies. J. Dairy Sci. 2009; 92:2057–2066.

[39] Leiber F., Kreuzer M., Nigg D., Wettstein HR., Scheeder MR. Lipids 2005; 40:191-202.

[40] Bartl K., Gomez CA., García M., Aufdermauer T., Kreuzer M., Hess HD., Wettstein HR. Milk fatty acid profile of Peruvian Criollo and Brown Swiss cows in response to different diet qualities fed at low and high altitude. Arch. Anim. Nutr. 2008; 62:468-484.

[41] Schroeder GF., Delahoy JE., Vidaurreta I., Bargo F., Gagliostro GA., Muller LD. Milk fatty acid composition of cows fed a total mixed ration or pasture plus concentrates replacing corn with fat. J. Dairy Sci. 2003; 86:3237-3248.

[42] Benchaar C., Peti, HV., Berthiaume R., Ouellet DR., Chiquette J., Chouinard PY. Effects of essential oils on digestion, ruminal fermentation, rumen microbial populations, milk production, and milk composition in dairy cows fed alfalfa silage or corn silage. J. Dairy Sci. 2007; 90:886-897.

[43] Chilliard Y., Ferlay A., Bernard L., Rouel J., Doreaue M., Diet, rumen biohydrogenation and nutritional quality of cow and goat milk fat. Eur. J. Lipid Sci. Technol. 2007; 109:828-855.

[44] Atroshi F., Rizzo A., Oestermann T., Parantainen J. Free fatty acids and lipid peroxidation in normal and mastitic bovine milk. J. Vet. Med. A 1989; 36:321-330.

[45] Miller RH., Bitman J., Bright SA., Wood DL., Capuco AV. Effect of clinical and subclinical mastitis on lipid composition of teat canal keratin. J. Dairy Sci. 1992; 75:1436-1442.

[46] Zhao X., Lacasse P. Mammary tissue damage during bovine mastitis: cause and control. J. Anim. Sci. 2008; 86 (Suppl 1) 57-65.

[47] Milne MH., Nolan AM., Cripps PJ., Fitzpatrick JL. Preliminary results of a study on pain assessment in clinical mastitis in dairy cows. In: Proceedings of the British Mastitis Conference Garstang, p117-119; 2003.

[48] Kemp MH., Nolan AM., Cripps PJ., Fitzpatrick JL. Animal-based measurements of the severity of mastitis in dairy cows. Vet. Rec. 2008; 163:175-179.

[49] Schrick FN., Hickett ME., Saxton AM., Lewis MJ., Dowlen HH., Olivers SP. Influence of subclinical mastitis during early lactation on reproductive parameters. J. Dairy Sci. 2001; 84:1407-1412.

[50] Groehn YT., Eicker SW., Ducrocq V., Hertl J.A. Effect of disease on the culling of Holstein dairy cows in New York State. J. Dairy Sci. 1998; 81:966-978.

[51] Caraviello DZ., Weigel KA., Shook GE., Ruegg PL. Assessment of the impact of somatic cell count on functional longevity in Holstein and Jersey cattle using survival analysis methodology. 2005; J. Dairy Sci. 88:804-811.

[52] Knaus W. Dairy cows trapped between performance demands and adaptability. J. Sci. Food Agric. 2009; 89:1107–1114.

[53] Hamann J. The impact of milking hygiene and management on mastitis. Bulletin of the Int Dairy Fed 2007; 416:25-33.

[54] Harmon RJ. Physiology of mastitis and factors affecting somatic cell counts. J. Dairy Sci. 1994; 77:2103-2112.

[55] Ma Y., Ryan C., Barbano DM., Galton DM., Rudgan MA., Boor KJ. Effects of somatic cell count on quality and shelf-life of pasteurized fluid milk. J. Dairy Sci. 2000; 83:264-274.

[56] Barbano DM., Ma, Y., Santos, MV. Influence of raw milk quality on fluid milk shelf life. J. Dairy Sci. 2006; 89:15-19.

[57] Lucey J. Cheesemaking from grass based seasonal milk and problems associated with late-lactation milk. J. Society of Dairy Techn. 1996; 49:59-64.

[58] O'Brian B., Gallagher B., Joyce P., Meaney WJ., Kelly A. Quality and safety of milk from farm to dairy product. www.teagasc.ie/research/reports/dairyproduction/4642/eopr-4642.pdf.; 1999.

[59] IDF (International Dairy Federation) Ann. Bull., part 3; 1967.

[60] IDF (International Dairy Federation) Bovine mastitis – Definitions and guidelines for diagnosis. IDF-Document 211; 1987.

[61] USDA (United States Department of Agriculture) (eds.) Somatic cell counts of milk from Dairy Herd Improvement herds during 2011. Animal Improvement Programs Laboratory, ARS-USDA, Beltsville, MD. In: https://aipl.arsusda.gov/publish/dhi/current/sccrpt.htm (accessed 23 August 2012).

[62] Hovi M., Sundrum A., Thamsborg SM. Animal health and welfare in organic livestock production in Europe: current state and future challenges. Livestock Production Science 2003; 80:41–53.

[63] Vaarst M., Leeb C., Nicholas P., Roderick S., Smolders G., Walkenhorst M., Brinkman J., March S., Stöger E., Gratzer E., Winckler C., Lund V., Henriksen BI., Hansen B., Neale M., Whistance L. Development of animal health and welfare planning in organic dairy farming in Europe. 16th IFOAM Organic World Congress; 2008.

[64] LeBlanc S., Lissemore K., Kelton D., Duffield T., Leslie K. Major advances in disease prevention in dairy cattle. J. Dairy Sci. 2006; 89:1267–1279.

[65] Valle P., Lien G., Flaten O., Koesling M., Ebbesvik M. Herd health and health management in organic versus conventional dairy herds in Norway. Livestock Science 2007; 112:123–132.

[66] Hardeng F., Edge V. Mastitis, ketosis, and milk fever in 31 organic and 93 conventional Norwegian dairy herds. J. Dairy Sci. 2001; 84:2673–2679.

[67] Sundberg T., Berglund B., Rydhmer L., Standberg E. Fertility, somatic cell count and milk production in Swedish organic and conventional dairy herds. Livestock Sience 2009; 126:176-182.

[68] Garmo R., Waage S., Sviland S., Henriksen BI., Osteras O., Reksen O. Reproductive Performance, Udder Health, and Antibiotic Resistance in Mastitis Bacteria isolated from Norwegian Red cows in Conventional and Organic Farming. Acta Vet Scand 2010; 52 (1) 11.

[69] Vaarst M., Bennedsgaard TW. Reduced Medication in Organic Farming with Emphasis on Organic Dairy Production. Acta Vet Scand 43 (Suppl 1) 51–57; 002.

[70] Hamilton C., Emanuelson U., Forslund K., Hansson I., Ekman T. Mastitis and related management factors in certified organic dairy herds in Sweden. Acta Vet Scand 2006; 48 (1) 11.

[71] Fall N., Emanuelson U., Martinsson K., Jonsson S. Udder health at a Swedish research farm with both organic and conventional dairy cow management. Preventive Veterinary Medicine 2008 a; 83:186–195.

[72] O'Mahony M., Healy A., O'Farrell K., Doherty M. Animal health and disease therapy on organic dairy farms in the republic of Ireland. Veterinary Record 2006; 159:680–682.

[73] Löf E., Gustafsson H., Emanuelson U. Associations between herd characteristics and reproductive efficiency in dairy herds. J. Dairy Sci. 2007; 90:4897–4907.

[74] Fall N., Gröhn Y., Forslund K., Essen-Gustafsson B., Niskanen R., Emanuelson U. An observational study on early-lactation metabolic profiles in Swedish organically and conventionally managed dairy cows. 2008 b; J. Dairy Sci. 91:3983–3992.

[75] Reksen O., Tverdal A., Ropstad E. A Comparative Study of Reproductive Performance in Organic and Conventional Dairy Husbandry. J. Dairy Sci. 1999; 82:2605–2610.

[76] Brinkmann J., Winckler, C. Animal health state in organic dairy farming-mastitis, lameness, metabolic disorders. In: Hess, J. and Rahmann, G. (eds.) Proceedings of the Scientific Conference on Organic Agriculture, 1.-4-. March, Kassel/Germany,; p343-346; 2005.

[77] Rutherford K., Langford F., Jack M., Sherwood L., Lawrence A., Haskell MJ. Lameness prevalence and risk factors in organic and non-organic dairy herds in the United Kingdom. The Veterinary Journal 2009; 180:95–105.

[78] Holzhauer M., Hardenberg C., Bartels C. Herd and cow-level prevalence of sole ulcers in The Netherlands and associated-risk factors. Preventive Veterinary Medicine 2009; 85:125–135.

[79] Kerestes M., Faigl V., Kulcsár M., Balogh O., Földi J., Fébel H., Chilliard Y., Huszenicza G. Periparturient insulin secretion and whole-body insulin responsiveness in dairy cows showing various forms of ketone pattern with or without puerperal metritis. Domestic Animal Endocrinology 2009; 37:250–261.

[80] Hardarson GH. Is the modern high potential dairy cow suitable for organic farming conditions? Acta Vetinaria Scandinavia 2001; Supplement 95: 63-67.

[81] Blanco-Penedo I., Fall I., Emanuelson U. Effects of turning to 100% organic feed on metabolic status of Swedish organic dairy cows. Livestock Science 2012; 143:242-248.

[82] Govasmark E., Steen A., Strøm T., Hansen S., Ram Singh B., Bernhoft A. Status of selenium and vitamin E on Norwegian organic sheep and dairy cattle farms. Acta Agriculturae Scandinavica, Section A - Animal Science 2005; 55:40–46.

[83] Ahlman T., Berglund B., Rydhmer L., Strandberg E. Culling reasons in organic and conventional dairy herds and genotype by environment interaction for longevity. J. Dairy Sci. 2011; 94:1568–1575.

[84] Thamsborg SM., Roderick S., Sundrum A. Animal Health and Diseases in Organic Farming: An overview, in: Vaarst M., Roderick S., Lund V., Lockeretz W. (Eds.), Animal Health and Welfare in Organic Agriculture. CAB International, p227–252; 2004.

[85] Sundrum A., Padel S., Arsenos G., Kuzniar A., Henriksen BI., Walkenhorst M., Vaarst M. Current and proposed EU legislation on organic livestock production with focus on animal health, welfare and food safety: a review, in: Rymer, C., Vaarst, M., Padel, S. (eds.), Future perspective for animal health on organic farms: main findings, conclusions and recommendations from SAFO Network Proceedings of the 5th SAFO Workshop,Odense, Denmark, p75–90; 2006.

[86] McInerney J. Old economics for new problems- livestock disease: Presidential address. Journal of Agricultural Economics 1996; 47:295–314.

[87] Sundrum A., Haerle C., Heissenhuber A. Udder health and farmer's income. Proceedings of the XIV ISAH-Congress 2009 (International Society of Animal Hygiene), 19th to 23rd July, Vechta, Germany, p119-122; 2009.

[88] Halasa T., Huijps K., Hogeveen H. Bovine mastitis, a review. Veterinary Quarterly 2007; 29:18–31.

[89] Hogeveen H. Costs of production diseases. Proceeding of the XXVII World Buiatrics Congress, p36-42; 2012.

[90] Huijps K., Hogeveen H., Lam TJ., Oude Lansink AJ. Costs and efficiacy of management measures to improve udder health on Dutch dairy farms. J. Dairy Sci. 2010; 93:115-124.

[91] Sundrum A. Conflicting areas in the ethical debate on animal health and welfare. In: Zollitsch, W., Winckler, C., Waiblinger, S., Halberger, A. (eds.), Sustainable food production and ethics. Wageningen Academic Publishers, p257-262; 2007.

[92] Kahnemann D. Thinking fast and slow. Penguin Books; 2011.

[93] Sundrum A. Udder health status on farm level –current state and perspectives from a systemic point of view. Berichte über Landwirtschaft 2010; 88:299-321.

[94] Sundrum A. Organic livestock production - trapped between aroused consumer expectations and limited resources. Proceedings of the 2nd Scientific Conference of the Int. Society of Organic Agriculture Research (ISOFAR) 18-20 June, Modena, Italy, p208-211; 2008.

Chapter 6

Organic and Conventional Farmers' Attitudes Towards Agricultural Sustainability

David Kings and Brian Ilbery

Additional information is available at the end of the chapter

http://dx.doi.org/10.5772/53072

1. Introduction

This chapter examines organic and conventional farmers' understandings of agricultural sustainability. Defined in the Brundtland Report as: 'development that meets the needs of the present without compromising the ability of future generations to meet their own needs' (World Commission on Environment and Development, 1987, p. 43), sustainability is a multi-faceted concept involving agronomic, ecological, economic, social and ethical considerations (Farshad & Zinck, 2003). It means different things to different people (Redclift, 1987; 1992 and O'Riordan, 1997). The focus in this chapter is specifically on the environmental dimensions of agricultural sustainability in the UK. Somewhat surprisingly, recent researchers have done little to engage critically with the concept of environmental sustainability. This may be because the socially and politically constructed concept is, according to Ilbery & Maye (2005), slippery and broad-ranging. However, this allows sustainability's fluid, constructed nature to be used more broadly and creatively (Maxey, 2007). It is now generally accepted that conventional farming systems have become environmentally unsustainable (Moore, 1962, 1966, 1970; Ratcliffe, 1962; Mellanby, 1967, 1970, 1981; Shoard, 1980; Burn, 2000; Pugliese, 2001; Storkey et al., 2011). Nevertheless, in late May 2012, Paul Christensen, chairman of the public body Natural England, said: 'I think we should embrace science [GM technology] that has increased [food] production'. This is in strict contrast to what the same body said in 2008, when it warned Gordon Brown not to rush headlong into GM crops (Gray, 2012). Such a change in emphasis reflects increasing concerns over food security, but it does raise issues over developing an agricultural system that is truly sustainable.

Aware of this dilemma, government policy in the UK now advocates the concept of sustainable intensification, which attempts to increase food production from the same area but without damaging the environment (Godfray et al., 2010; Lang & Barling, 2012). Supporters of this approach claim that substantial increases in crop yield can be provided through science and technology. Examples include crop improvement, more efficient use of water and fertilizers, the introduction of new non-chemical approaches to crop protection, the reduction of post-harvest losses and more sustainable livestock (Maye & Ilbery, 2011). However, it is debatable whether sustainable intensification can be achieved without significant increases in the use of chemical inputs, leading Lang & Barling (2012) to describe the concept as an oxymoron.

In contrast, organic farming is a holistic production management system that promotes and enhances agro-ecosystem health, including biodiversity, biological cycles and soil biological activity. It also emphasises the use of management practices, in preference to the use of off-farm inputs, and recognises that regional conditions require locally-adapted systems (Codex Alimentarius Commission, 1999). In March 2008, the World Board of the International Federation of Organic Agriculture Movements (IFOAM) approved the following definition: 'Organic agriculture is a production system that sustains the health of soils, ecosystems and people. It relies on ecological processes, biodiversity and cycles adapted to local conditions, rather than the use of inputs with adverse effects. Organic agriculture combines tradition, innovation and science to benefit the shared environment and promote fair relationships and good quality of life for all involved'.

There are many different organic farming practices, each with its diverse views of nature and value assumptions. They involve a variety of alternative methods of agricultural production which evolve as new scientific research becomes available. However, they retain a fundamental philosophical perspective of working with, not dominating, natural systems and having respect for the natural environment (Lampkin, 1990; Fuller, 1997; Guthman, 2004). While some writers are concerned that organic farming systems are becoming 'conventionalised' in their production, marketing and distribution methods (Buck et al., (1997; Lockie & Halpin, 2005; Rosin & Campbell, 2009), others feel that they have the potential to 'develop in distinct ways in different national contexts' (Hall & Mogyorody, 2001, p. 401; see also Coombes & Campbell, 1998 and Guthman, 2004).

Provision of adequate water supplies is a key requirement for the sustainability of organic and conventional farming, the UK's two dominant agricultural systems. But, according to Edward-Jones & Howells (2001), there is no absolute and available measure of sustainability. Thus it is debatable which of these two farming systems is the more sustainable, although organic farming is more so in a bio-physical sense (Edward-Jones & Howells, 2001). Of course, extreme climatic events can have potentially serious consequences for agricultural sustainability, as demonstrated in the early months of 2012 in the UK. While the most severe water shortage since 1976 was reported in March 2012, April was the wettest month on record (Hall, 2012a and b).

Farming itself, through the use of fertilisers, fuel and methane produced by livestock, has the potential to adversely affect agricultural sustainability through increases in global temperatures. Climate change also poses the single greatest long-term threat to birds (RSPB, 2011), which have been used as significant indicator species of the environmental health and

http://dx.doi.org/10.5772/53072

sustainability of agriculture since the early-1960s (Moore, 1962; Moore & Ratcliffe, 1962; Ratcliffe, 1963; Moore & Walker, 1964).

This chapter explores in further detail some of the key issues affecting the environmental dimensions of agricultural sustainability in the UK. More specifically, it uses an essentially behavioural approach to compare the perceptions and attitudes of those farmers loosely labelled 'organic' and 'conventional' towards environmental aspects of agricultural sustainability. The chapter has the following two interrelated objectives:

- To evaluate farmers' environmental perceptions, attitudes and behaviour towards organic farming and the development of more environmentally sustainable farming practices.
- To assess different environmental understandings of organic and conventional farmers, located in central-southern England, towards selected themes relating to environmental dimensions of agricultural sustainability.

The rest of the chapter is divided into four sections. The next section reviews some important dimensions of behavioural approaches to research. This is followed by a description of the 'extensive' and 'intensive' research methodologies adopted in the investigation. Section four provides insights into some farm and farmer characteristics, investigates farmers' perceptions and attitudes towards some key issues relating to agricultural sustainability, and examines farmers' contextual life histories and work routines. A final section provides a conclusion to the chapter.

2. Behavioural approaches

Morris & Potter (1995) defined behavioural studies as: '... one which focuses on the motives, values and attitudes that determine the decision-making process of individual farmers'. According to Wood (2000), although attitudes may remain constant over time and context, they do not directly explain behaviour because attitudes can be arrived at from different experiences. Behavioural approaches allow for the recognition of farmers as independent environmental managers who often make decisions about the management of resources on their farms independent from the state or other 'official' environmental managers. The focus on individual decision makers, together with the possibility of formulating interview-based research methodologies, are key reasons why behavioural approaches have been adopted by researchers endeavouring to 'understand' the decision making of farmers (Wilson, 1997). According to Beedell & Rehman (1999), such methodologies can be standardised and repeatable, thereby making them useful in monitoring change over time for EU policy-makers. These requirements have contributed to a recent increase in the application of 'behavioural approaches' to investigate issues such as food security and agricultural sustainability. Nevertheless, behavioural approaches which use inflexible structured questionnaire methodologies and focus on individual decision makers out of their social or familial milieus may appear elementary in attempting to understanding human behaviour (Burton, 2004). In order to alleviate such problems, Burton (2004) suggested combining quantitative and qualitative work in behavioural research.

The classic behavioural approach refers to a broad range of studies that employ actor-oriented quantitative methodologies in the investigation of decision-making (Burton, 2004). Although criticised for their relative neglect of 'spatial science' and 'partial' treatment of people (Cloke et al., 1991), behavioural perspectives have been used widely in agricultural research (Wolpert, 1964; Gasson, 1973, 1974; Gillmor, 1986; Ilbery, 1978, 1985; Brotherton, 1990; Morris & Potter, 1995; Wilson, 1996, 1997; Beedell & Rehman, 1999, 2000; Burton, 2004; Kings & Ilbery, 2010, 2011) and successfully applied to the examination and understandings of farmers' environmental behaviours. Farmers make their environmental decisions as they perceive it, not as it is, but the action resulting from their decision is played out in a real environment (Brookfield, 1969). Behavioural approaches are appropriate for examining the perception/cognition, values, attitudes and opinions of farmers and how they relate to environmental dimensions of agricultural sustainability (see Kings & Ilbery (2011) for details of how perception/cognition relate to farmers' attitudes and behaviours).

This chapter adopts 'extensive' and 'intensive' approaches to the examination of organic and conventional farmers' attitudes, values and behaviours toward environmental components of agricultural sustainability. Lowland farmland bird populations are used as a key indicator of farmers' environmental awareness, concerns, attitudes and behaviours. An important reason for using farmland avifauna in this way relates to the Department for Environment, Food and Rural Affairs (Defra) use of wild bird population trends as a 'headline indicator' of the 'sustainability' of its policies and 'quality of life' in the UK (Anon, 1999).

Four key and linked areas of farmers' understandings of environmental aspects of agricultural sustainability are advocated in this study: 'responsible' behaviour, uptake of environmental schemes, readership of agricultural publications and conservation work. One may expect differences in each of these between organic and conventional farmers. For example, while conventional farmers may perceive responsible behaviour as keeping the land in a good, fertile condition for growing crops and raising livestock, organic farmers may espouse concerns for protecting the land from environmental degradation. Likewise, one might expect organic farmers to be more interested in joining environmental schemes such as Countryside Stewardship and LEAF. This, in turn, might reflect the reading of different agricultural journals and magazines, as well as different attitudes towards conservation work, with perhaps organic farmers engaging more in pond, hedge and woodland creation and conventional farmers in creating pheasant cover.

3. A methodological framework

The methodology used for examining farmers' characteristics and attitudes towards the four environmental components of agricultural sustainability themes was in two distinct stages. Stage one consisted of hour-long telephone interviews with twenty-five organic farmers and twenty-five conventional farmers – located in central-southern England. Most farmers can be contacted by telephone, although they may not be listed in business or private telephone directories. Organic farmers, selected from the official regional Soil Association and Organic Farmers and Growers membership lists, were interviewed first. Each respondent was asked to provide details of a local conventional farmer who they thought was appropriate for interview. This method provided dependable geographically linked pairs of farmers during the investigation. The study was limited to farms/farmers in central-southern England. Any concerns about providing a reliable national representative sample were unwarranted as it was anticipated that the sample may or may not be representative of farms and farmers in the UK as a whole. A questionnaire was designed for use in the 'extensive' data gathering approach. These data were analysed both quantitatively, using summarising statistics, and qualitatively, in the form of farmers' quotations and illustrative farm cameos to emphasise the arguments being developed about environmental dimensions of agricultural sustainability. This analysis was used to support, illustrate and broaden the statistical data related to farm/farmer characteristics. The resulting similarities and differences between the two study groups provided environmental insights into their behaviour in relation to agricultural sustainability.

Stage two of the methodology consisted of 3 hour on-farm intensive qualitative/ interpretive interviews, with five geographically linked pairs of organic and conventional farmers who, earlier in the investigation, had been involved in the extensive telephone survey. It is important to note that the reference codes assigned to the ten respondents in section 4.3 are not always the same as those used in sections 4.1 and 4.2. The organic farmers were coded OF1 to OF5 and the conventional respondents CF1 to CF5 to facilitate data analysis. An illustrative sample of different ages, farm holdings of different sizes and systems was selected in preference to a representative sample. An interview guide was designed which also prompted respondents to talk about their life histories and work routines. The interviews were recorded using a Digital Audio MiniDisc-recorder with stereo microphone and transcribed soon after for analysis. In contrast to the extensive telephone survey, the data generated from stage two of the methodology were analysed using a textual approach using words and meanings. Any interesting or unusual quotations and paraphrases made by respondents were analysed in order to demonstrate attitudinal similarities and differences. The interviews produced contextual findings relating to the respondents' environmental understandings and behaviours towards agricultural sustainability which provided a broad picture of environmental dimensions of agricultural sustainability in central-southern England.

In the next section, the adopted 'extensive' and 'intensive' research methodology will be used primarily to examine and gain insights into the perceptions, values, opinions and behaviours of organic and conventional farmers in relation to their awareness and understandings of environmental dimensions of agricultural sustainability.

4. Examining farmers' attitudes and behaviours

The behavioural approach is used first, to examine farm and farmer characteristics; second, to examine the attitudes, understandings and behaviours of organic and conventional farmers (located in central-southern England) in relation to environmental dimensions of agricultural sustainability; and third, to ascertain if farmers' attitudes and behaviours support those expressed earlier in the analysis.

4.1. Contrasting organic and conventional farms and farmers

The analysis began with an examination of farm/farmer characteristics of the 50 telephone interviewees as they are likely to influence farmers' relationship with the four core themes related to environmental aspects of agricultural sustainability. A number of significant similarities and differences were found in terms of farm/farmer characteristics during the extensive organic and conventional farmer telephone survey. First, conventional farms (average size 202.3ha) were larger than organic farms (average size 85.4ha), although the size of both farm types was extremely variable (see Table 1).

		Organic farmers			Conventional farmers		
Hectares	**Acres**	**Frequency**	**%**	**Mean ha**	**Frequency**	**%**	**Mean ha**
0-40	0-100	14	56	15.57	2	8	36.5
42-202	101-500	9	36	91.44	17	68	107.53
203-405	501-1000	1	4	364	3	12	296.33
406-810	1001-2000	1	4	730	2	8	526
"/>810	"/>2000	0	0	0	1	4	1133
Total		25	100		25	100	

Table 1. Distribution of sampled organic and conventional farms

Secondly, if cereals were grown on any of the organic farms, they were usually used as livestock fodder or seed. This study was in accord with Ilbery et al's, (1999) findings that in national terms central-southern England is a marginal cereal production area. Grass and fodder enterprises associated with organic livestock were the most common organic types found on the surveyed organic farms. Lampkin (1990) notes that grassland is often the most trouble-free and least expensive land to convert to organic production. Inorganic fertiliser applications to conventional grassland is incompatible with the maintenance of biological diversity (Sotherton & Self, 2000). Within the context of this chapter, biodiversity, as it is commonly referred to, is defined as the variation of plant and animal life at a respondent's farm. A key priority facing agricultural sustainability is the protection of the environment and natural resources such as water, soil and biodiversity (Defra, 2006). Biodiversity is therefore essential for maintaining agricultural sustainability. According to Willer & Gillmor (1992), many farmers experiment with organic grassland production before deciding to convert their whole farm to organic production. This contrasted with more arable crops being grown on conventional farms. Thirdly, a wide range of livestock was found on the organic farms such as chickens, pigs, cattle (beef and dairy cows), sheep, goats and deer, with some organic farmers having up to four different animal species. In contrast, dairy cattle, beef cattle or sheep were usually the norm on the conventional farms.

Fourthly, more organic than conventional farms were owner-occupied. This is linked to the first key point that organic farms tend to be smaller than conventional farms and, subject to other influencing factors such as land quality and location, may therefore be less expensive. Organic farms are also more diverse in their enterprises thereby providing greater levels of biodiversity and agricultural sustainability, in contrast to the greater size dictated by specialisation. Fifthly, more than three times as many conventional as organic farmers were of mixed tenure. This may be partially explained by these conventional farmers renting additional land with a view to obtaining significant economies of scale; for example, as required by monocultures in the cultivation of GM crops which are considered by many researchers to be unsustainable.

Finally, the two survey groups had similar numbers of vocational qualifications, although organic farmers had the highest number of qualifications towards the upper end of the education spectrum (Table 2). Examining qualifications relating specifically to agriculture shows that more conventional than organic farmers have a national certificate in agriculture. In contrast, only the organic farmers have a higher degree or Doctorate.

	Organic		Conventional	
	Frequency	**Percentage**	**Frequency**	**Percentage**
Certificate	1	4	0	0
National Cert in Agriculture	1	4	5	20
Ordinary Diploma	3	12	2	8
Higher Diploma	0	0	2	8
Degree	6	24	1	4
Higher Degree	2	8	0	0
Doctorate	1	4	0	0
None	11	44	15	60
Total	**25**	**100**	**25**	**100**

It should be noted that only the highest qualification awarded to each farmer has been used in this table.

Table 2. Qualifications obtained by farmers

To gain insights into farmers' attitudes towards environmental dimensions of the core agricultural sustainability theme, 'responsible countryside behaviour', respondents were asked how farmers should 'behave' in the countryside. The term 'behave responsibly' was used more by organic than conventional farmers. Organic farmers also used words such as 'stewards, keepers, custodians or protectors', contrasting with conventional farmers who preferred to use the words 'looking after, care and good condition'. This highlights an important difference between the two survey groups. While conventional farmers understand responsible countryside behaviour as having tidy farms with neatly trimmed hedges and weed-free fields through herbicide usage, organic respondents' understanding and implementation of the term is untidy farms with 'over grown' hedges and less attention paid to removing weeds. The latter farming practices result in greater levels of biodiversity, essential for agricultural sustainability, than on the conventional farms.

The actual countryside behaviour of respondents was examined by asking four related questions directly linked to four specific environmental dimensions of agricultural sustainability: first, membership of agri-environmental schemes; second, participation in conservation work; third, membership of environmental organisations; and fourth, 'readership' of agri-environmental journals and magazines.

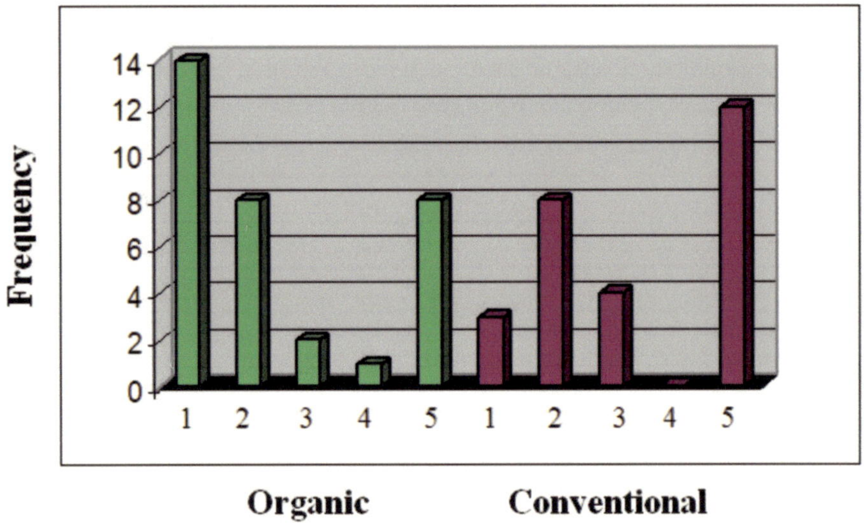

Figure 1. Farmers' uptake of agri-environmental schemes. 1 = Countryside Stewardship Scheme; 2 = Set-aside Scheme; 3 = Environmentally Sensitive Areas; 4 = Linking Environment and Farming; 5 = None

The data in Figure 1 suggest that organic farmers are more interested in joining agri-environmental schemes than conventional farmers. Many more organic than conventional farmers belong to more than one scheme. In excess of half of the organic farmers were in the Countryside Stewardship Scheme, contrasting with just over one tenth of conventional farmers. The Countryside Stewardship was the government's main scheme for countryside until the introduction of Environmental Stewardship. Farmers entered 10-year agreements to manage land in an environmentally sustainable way in return for annual payments (Defra, 2002). There were equal numbers of both types of farmer involved with the set-aside scheme which has played an important role in biodiversity and agricultural sustainability.

http://dx.doi.org/10.5772/53072

Some interesting differences emerged between the two survey groups concerning the type of conservation work carried out by farmers (see Table 3). First, more organic than conventional farmers undertake conservation work, with a much higher proportion involved in hedge laying and wood planting demonstrating their ecocentic attitudes. Secondly, conventional farmers see the creation of pheasant cover as conservation works and nearly 1 in 4 do not undertake any kind of conservation work. Conservation work, particularly the recreation of ponds, woods and hedges by some organic farmers, plays a vital role in helping to restore agricultural sustainability to pre intensification levels.

	Organic farmers		Conventional farmers	
	Frequency	**%**	**Frequency**	**%**
Don't do conservation work	1	4	6	24
On-farm conservation	24	96	19	76
Off-farm conservation - voluntary/ Contract	3	12	0	0
Hedges: planting, laying and restoration	19	76	4	16
Woodland: plant, coppice and pollard	15	60	4	16
Ponds: create and maintain	6	24	3	12
Meadows: plant and maintain	5	20	4	16
Pheasant cover	0	0	4	16
Totals	**24**	**96**	**19**	**76**

Table 3. Frequency of farmers carrying out conservation work

Membership of environmental institutions was quite low among both groups of farmers. But, differences did emerge which reflected attitudes towards conservation work and environmental components of agricultural sustainability. Thus, while organic farmers preferred the Wildlife Trust, Woodland Trust and Friends of the Earth, conventional farmers usually preferred the Game Conservancy Trust. This raises the important question about how 'green' such environmental agencies actually are. The most frequently mentioned agency was the Game Conservancy Trust, which was dominated by conventional farmers whose main countryside leisure pursuit is shooting.

Further significant differences between organic and conventional farmers were found in relation to the readership of magazines and journals. Thus, while *Farmers Weekly* and, to a much less extent, *Farmers Guardian* were the most popular conventional farmers' reading, the *Living Earth* and *Organic Farming* were read most widely among organic farmers. The periodicals preferred by the organic respondents were primarily concerned with environmental and sustainability issues other than agriculture. The most popular magazine overall by far was the *Farmers Weekly*. Generally, organic farmers seemed more critical in their reading habits than conventional respondents. These findings reflected the earlier differences between the two groups of farmers in terms of membership of environmental organisations and agri-environmental schemes. It is not surprising, therefore, that considerable differences in perceptions, attitudes and understandings emerged in relation to the closely linked environmental dimensions of agricultural sustainability concepts.

4.2. Exploring environmental dimensions of agricultural sustainability

Section one introduced six environmental concepts related to the core theme of agricultural sustainability. These, in order of least environmentally acceptable to most acceptable, are:

- Global climate change and extreme weather events
- Genetically Modified crops
- United Kingdom and European Union agricultural policy
- Conventional agriculture
- Organic farming systems
- Lowland farmland avifauna

A number of wide ranging differences of opinion were found between many of the interviewees towards the related environmental dimensions of agricultural sustainability concepts during the following farmer discussions which may shape their attitudes towards agricultural sustainability. For example, a number of organic farmers believed that global climate change is caused by burning fossil fuels and they suggested some resulting agricultural changes such as growing new varieties of crops:

'Well global climate change is going to have a profound effect on agriculture. The worst predictions suggest that all countries will have to grow different crops' (OF1).

In contrast, several conventional farmers thought that changes in weather patterns are part of the normal course of events. Historically, climate has always changed and is therefore likely to do so in the future. Some researchers, similar to conventional farmers, suggest that fear of global warming derives from politics and dogma rather than scientific proof (Plimer, 2009). Global climate change is a particularly important issue because it has the potential to reduce provision of water supplies, as discussed earlier, so essential for the sustainability of organic and conventional agriculture. However, not all extreme weather events have such potentially negative effects on agricultural sustainability. At the time of writing (30th June 2012), it was announced by the Environment Agency that there had been more rainfall for late spring and early summer than at any time since 1910, when the first readings were made. Nearly half of the rivers the Environment Agency monitors are at exceptionally high levels, with all rivers higher than, or at normal levels for the time of the year (Alleyne, 2012). But, earlier this year, crop failure was occurring widely due to extreme drought conditions. More recently, 'excessive' widespread flooding has also resulted in large-scale crop failure. Both types of 'extreme' weather event have proved to be detrimental for environmental components of agricultural sustainability.

Equally harmful, most organic farmers in the survey believed that government policy had caused a lot of damage to the countryside thereby reducing biodiversity and agricultural sustainability, typically stating: '... grubbing out hedges was a mistake' (OF11). In contrast, most conventional farmers said that the damage to the countryside was minimal, typically commenting: 'I suppose some places where the water comes from you have to be a bit careful with nitrates and things ...' (CF10). Conventional farmers seemed to have more faith than organic farmers in the government's willingness to rectify such past environmental damage to the countryside, typically commenting: 'Yes, they [the government] are under pressure by the public to do so' (CF25). Many more conventional than organic farmers (16-2) claimed that there is an important relationship between government and environmental issues, characterised by comments such as: 'I think the government has become anti-farming – they are doing more and more for the environment and cutting back on agriculture' (CF4). In contrast, twice as many organic as conventional farmers thought that: 'This present government is not getting more environmentally friendly' (OF18). The attitudes revealed by the above comments indicate that most organic respondents have greater levels of environmental concern for their farms than many of the conventional farmers.

Another important concern of many organic farmers is the perceived environmental problems associated with GM technology, typically commenting: 'I see no situation, with our present knowledge of GM, where it would give environmental benefits – you are asking for trouble – I can't see any sensible person agreeing with it being a good thing' (OF20). This contrasted with most conventional farmers who seemed a little more accepting of GM technology than the organic respondents, typically saying: 'I haven't a huge fear of them as long as we observe the science ...' (CF24). Conventional farmers were generally less critical of GM crops than the organic respondents, and seem to place their main emphasis on the potential environmental benefits to be gained from reductions in pesticide use. However, one organic respondent raised the issue that GM crops are associated with monocultures. Monocultures are generally unsuitable for many lowland farmland birds as they may have to rely on fewer prey species, particularly during adverse weather conditions. In contrast, on most arable organic farms birds are able to move to alternative food-bearing habitats. A consequence of such intensive farming methods is the loss of the incidental habitats, often associated with organic farming, which reduces biodiversity and thus agricultural sustainability.

Many organic farmers were equally concerned about the environmental sustainability of conventional farming. For example, more than 50 per cent organic farmers said that conventional agriculture is harmful to the environment and therefore unsustainable. Several gave specific reasons for their environmental concern such as conventional farmers using high levels of nitrate and pesticides on crops. This contrasted with many conventional farmers who were less likely to believe that conventional agriculture is having negative environmental impacts. Almost all organic farmers were critical of conventional respondents in the way in which conventional agriculture damages water quality through pesticides usage. Such practices are likely to have a detrimental effect on future agricultural sustainability. Organic respondents' attitudes towards this issue were epitomised by comments such as: 'I definitely think it [conventional agriculture] has a negative effect on water quality'. In contrast, only 40 per cent of conventional farmers said that conventional agriculture is harmful to water quality and a further twenty per cent said that conventional agriculture didn't affect water quality, with quotes like: 'pesticides – it doesn't make any difference'.

At the other end of the spectrum, the surveyed organic farmers were very critical of pesticide use which can reduce biodiversity and thus agricultural sustainability. This contrasted with conventional farmers, who believed they need to use pesticides to produce their crops but, nevertheless, are aware of the dangers of over-use of such chemicals. Typical organic farmers' responses included: 'Conventional farming is lazy farming; it's farming out of a can, whereas with organic farming, you have to farm with your head' (OF2). Other organic farmers were more detailed with their response, such as the 54 year old owner/tenant organic farmer who said:

'If you read the magazine that the conventional farmers read, the *Farmers Weekly*, you will notice that the magazine is paid for by pesticide adverts. The biggest adverts saying this is the time to spray with this or that. This is the way [conventional] farmers are being educated' (OF5).

Some conventional farmers agreed with organic farmers that conventionally produced crops sometimes use high levels of pesticides; however, they tended to justify their position by typically saying: 'I think that we are forced by economics to using and growing the things [crops] the best we can – if we want to be farmers we have to do it that way' (CF24).

In contrast to their understandings that conventional farming is unsustainable, almost three quarters of organic respondents thought that organic agriculture is environmentally sustainable. A number of independent studies support that viewpoint (Morgan & Murdoch, 2000; Hansen et al., 2001; Lotter, 2003; Darnhofer, 2005; Kings & Ilbery, 2010; 2011). This contrasted with the conventional farmers who were generally not in support of those views, typified by the following comment: 'I think organic grass farmers cause more problems with nitrates than I do by ploughing clover [into their soil]' (CF13). Interestingly, one in two organic respondents claimed environmental concerns to be their main reason for adoption of organic methods and a further twenty per cent thought they had always farmed organically. Such comments reveal their ecocentric attitudes towards agricultural sustainability. Significantly, half of those who emphasised environmental reasons had a degree or higher degree, possibly suggesting a link between higher education and environmental awareness.

It emerged that most of the organic respondents believed that organic arable farmers use a lot of fossil fuels in their mechanical weeding processes, as typified by this comment: 'The burners they use I would think they use a colossal amount of fuel' (OF2). This practice contributes to climate warming and is therefore liable to have a detrimental effect on long-term agricultural sustainability through reduced crop yield and/or failure. This finding does not support the belief that organic farming systems are always environmentally sustainable. It is noteworthy that several organic respondents declined to comment, possibly because they were aware that more fossil fuels are used in mechanical weeding processes than chemical methods of weeding. Interestingly, most conventional farmers in the survey did not disapprove of organic farmers regarding this issue.

http://dx.doi.org/10.5772/53072

Lowland farmland bird populations are strongly influenced by all of the above environmental dimensions of agricultural sustainability. The analysis therefore attempts to draw together some of these closely related concepts through an examination of respondents' attitudes, beliefs and awareness of lowland farmland avifauna. The first loosely worded question asked respondents how they thought modern agriculture relates to farmland birds, thereby enabling answers which could relate to any of the previous linked concepts such as conventional farming. The core point to emerge from the analysis was that organic respondents believe organic farming systems are 'better' for birds than conventional agriculture, typified by the following comment: 'This is just a small organic dairy farm and it's full of birds but I work on another farm [as a contractor], which is an intensive dairy farm and there's no birds on it' (OF7). However, some conventional farmers, whilst acknowledging that intensive farming has been harmful to birds in the past, tended to justify the current population levels and mix of farmland avifauna by blaming government agri-environmental policy for reducing agricultural sustainability: 'There are fewer birds now [on lowland farmland] because farmers have been forced out of mixed farming systems' (CF1).

Similar to earlier discussions regarding government policy, the majority of members of both groups of respondents had little faith that the government would be successful in its aim of restoring farmland bird populations to sustainable 1970 levels by 2020. Organic farmers typically commented: '2020 is a frightfully convenient date – it's the sort of date that governments love – it's well into the future and people have short memories' (OF1). Equally as cynical, typical conventional respondents' comments included: 'Not if they [the government] put a ban on hunting and shooting – there are too many pests – I kill 80-100 Carrion Crows and Magpies each year' (CF1). It seems unlikely that the population of corvids will remain sustainable in CF1's farm location if he continues with his current attitudes and patterns of behaviour. Importantly, it may be that climatic factors have been overlooked in the distribution of birds by other influences, such as the alteration of habitats, for example, as caused through the intensification of agriculture. Recent anecdotal evidence suggests that farmland birds have had a very poor 2012 breeding season due to extremely high rainfall levels noted earlier. Generally, the attitudes and behaviours of organic farmers suggest a more a sustainable approach than the conventional respondents towards lowland farmland avifauna, which are used as significant indicator species of the environmental health and sustainability of agriculture.

4.3. On-farm intensive qualitative interviews

Farmers' contextual life histories and work routines were examined to ascertain if these helped to explain some of the results revealed in sections 4.1 and 4.2 regarding concerns related to environmental components of agricultural sustainability.

Contextual life histories and work routines

Although the ten separate descriptive farmer contextual life histories, obtained from the intensive farm interviews, may not be representative of conventional and organic farmers generally, examination of their life histories and the way in which they relate to farming and the farm environment revealed some thought-provoking insights into their environmental attitudes, beliefs and behaviours towards environmental dimensions of agricultural sustainability. Most of the conventional respondents seemed to place great importance on their early work experience on other farms and saw this as a crucial building block from which they have developed their own particular 'style' of farming. This experience was common to respondents CF3, CF4 and CF5, and typified by respondent CF3 who finished school aged fifteen: ' ... the best thing I did was going round a multitude of farms working for other people, because you see how different people tackle the same job from a different angle'. OF1 also considered that his early on-farm practical experiences influenced his farming philosophy: 'those early years spent almost entirely outside doing physical work must have been formative and very important to me'. A common denominator of these four farmers is that they all started in farming at a young age without formal qualifications, although OF1 and CF5 gained a National Diploma in Agriculture when older. As discussed in the previous section, independent research shows that environmental concern for issues related to agricultural sustainability was correlated with variables such as age and education.

Another important insight to emerge from the life histories is that the conventional respondents' idea of agriculture was often well-organised, neat and tidy farms with the land in 'good shape', as epitomised by CF1, CF3 and CF4. This was illustrated by CF1 who, when seeing litter, would stop his truck to collect it. CF3 also demonstrated his extreme tidiness by apologising for failing to remove what appeared to be the last remnant of scrub so essential for farm biodiversity and, ultimately, productive, wildlife friendly and sustainable agriculture. These attitudes and on-farm behaviours contrasted significantly with respondents OF1 and OF4's high level of environmental concern and seemingly less tidy approach to farming. According to CF4, his sister (OF4): 'is a muddler ... a policeman said to somebody [about her dwelling] I would never know whether it's been burgled or not'. These attitudes and behaviours support the earlier findings towards the core environmental dimension of agricultural sustainability theme 'responsible countryside behaviour', which showed that conventional farmers' often have tidy farms, neatly trimmed hedges and fields kept weed-free through herbicide usage. This contrasted with organic farmers' untidy farms with 'over grown' hedges and less concern about removing weeds, with their associated invertebrates and weed seeds, which contribute significantly towards increased levels of biodiversity, an important environmental components of agricultural sustainability.

Several of the conventional farmers showed technocentric attitudes. According to O'Riordan (1981), technocentrism is a mode of thought which recognises environmental problems but believes that society will always solve them through technology and achieve unlimited material growth. This contrasted with the more ecocentric attitudes of some of the organic respondents. Ecocentricism can be defined as a mode of thought which regards humans as subject to ecological and system laws; essentially it is not human-centred (anthropocentric) but centred on natural ecosystems, of which humans are just another component (O'Riordan, 1981). A final insight to emerge was that most of the organic respondents planted hedges and created ponds, thereby directly contributing to biodiversity and agricultural sustainability. Organic farmers also had a vision of farming more closely linked to the 'natural' environment than several of the conventional farmers, whose concept of 'nature' was re-

http://dx.doi.org/10.5772/53072

lated to planting pheasant cover and providing 'good environments' for foxes. CF1 claimed to be a keen naturalist and countryman and recalls happy childhood memories of: '... shooting rabbits and squirrels with a 410 hammer gun'. These findings support the results from the examination of the core theme of farmers' conservation work where it was found that more organic than conventional farmers undertake conservation work, with many carrying out hedge laying, pond creation and wood planting. This type of habitat creation plays an important role in helping to restore agricultural sustainability to pre intensification levels. In contrast, conventional farmers are more likely to see the creation of pheasant cover as conservation work.

Having gained some further insights into the five geographically linked organic and conventional farmers' environmental perceptions, attitudes and behaviours, the examination turns to farmers' work routines which may reveal additional insights into environmental dimensions of agricultural sustainability. Respondents' work routines revolved around the recurring times of seasons, the cycles of planting and harvesting of crops, and the cycles of birth and death of livestock and ultimately people. However, organic farmers' work routine was usually more complex than the conventional case study respondents due to the diversity of their enterprises. This supports the earlier findings in the farmer characteristics section. Many respondents' work patterns were built around their livestock; for example, specialist dairy farmer CF2's work routine was dictated throughout the whole year by milking his cows twice a day. He sees himself as a producer of 'good English food [milk] for the housewife.' Similarly, a mixed farmer's comments seem to set in stone the inflexibility of his work routine: 'It's the dairy herd we have to milk twice a day, so that's it – all year round' (CF3), although this situation would be equally true of an organic dairy farm. CF1's daily activities revolved around his flock of 1,000 ewes; however, this work routine was disrupted when a ram could not be restrained.

Some farmers claimed their work routine is very tiring. The often exhausting seasonal work was epitomised by a mixed organic respondent who kept a wide range of livestock on her farm, including fish in a recently excavated lake thereby increasing biodiversity levels on her holding. She illustrated some of the complexities of her daily work routine by detailing several aspects of a 'typically' tiring day during the lambing season:

'Parts of my routine are seasonal. It usually starts at six thirty, but at half past three this morning I was still trugging away getting a lamb to feed. I had one lamb that we saved whose eyes were pecked out by a crow, but it hadn't healed properly and it went straight into joint ill and died' (OF2).

This description demonstrated vividly the rhythm of life and death on her farm and showed her individual care and attention to livestock. She emphasised the importance of feeding her animals with natural healthy food to ensure their good health.

The diversity of OF4's holding and the size, type and biodiversity of her farm's hilly terrain strongly influenced her work routine. Her contextual life history revealed that, in contrast to the other organic respondents, she had off-farm jobs thereby adding to the complexity of her daily work routine. Her brother's (CF4) weekday work pattern revolved principally around three issues: first, his non-farming duties with his children because his wife works full time as a teacher; second, early morning feeding and moving his sheep between fields as necessary and; third, having a regular shoot in the pheasant cover he created. This supports the earlier findings that conventional farmers often see the creation of pheasant cover as conservation works.

The weekday work pattern of OF1 was strongly influenced by the limitations on the amount of time he can work at any one period, due to his serious illness which requires eating and resting at frequent intervals: 'My work routine revolves around my illness – I have had ME for seventeen years and can only work for short periods then I have to have a rest' (OF1). In line with other farmers, he said his work pattern was dictated by the seasons and he used words such as 'revolves' which indicate a cyclical pattern of time. He claimed that his farming practices were 'based on nature and natural processes which work best on their own', thereby further revealing his ecocentric attitudes and behaviours.

Initially, it seemed surprising that all the respondents focused on the daily routine of looking after livestock when some are mixed farmers; however, this may indicate that the immediacy and care required by farm animals is considered more important than, in the short term, raising crops. Many of the quotations demonstrated the cyclical nature of farming as a common thread linking all farmers. However, the organic farmers seemed to have a significantly closer relationship with their livestock than conventional respondents, which may simply be due to them caring for smaller numbers of animals; however, other factors such as the life experiences of OF2 as a nurse and her ecocentric attitudes may also be important.

The attitudes and behaviours of both groups of respondents during their work routines helped support earlier findings towards environmental dimensions of agricultural sustainability. This was epitomised by some organic farmers' individual concern for their stock and considerable interest in carrying out conservation work. This often contrasted significantly with some of the conventional farmers' who showed little interest in conservation work other than related to shooting.

5. Conclusion

This chapter used an essentially behavioural approach to examine the environmental attitudes, understandings and behaviours of organic and conventional farmers (in central-southern England) towards four core agricultural sustainability themes and a range of supporting and interrelated environmental dimensions of agricultural sustainability concepts. Whether loosely labelled organic or conventional, a diverse series of environmental perceptions, attitudes and behaviours emerged from the respondents. For example, in terms of 'responsible countryside behaviour', conventional farmers tended to have tidy farms with neatly trimmed hedges and weed-free fields, with the aim of maintaining their land in good, fertile condition. Burton (2004) also noted that: 'a number of researchers found that conventional farmers have a penchant for landscapes that are neat, clean and ordered'. In contrast, organic respondents generally had relatively untidy farms with 'over grown' hedges and

http://dx.doi.org/10.5772/53072

paid considerably less attention to removing weeds. Both of these play important roles in the biodiversity element of agricultural sustainability. Organic farmers were also more interested in joining environmental schemes than conventional farmers, with many belonging to more than one scheme, particularly those associated with the 'natural' environment such as Countryside Stewardship and LEAF. However, similar numbers of organic and conventional respondents were in a set-aside scheme, which later proved to be of great benefit for agricultural sustainability through increased biodiversity. However, many conventional farmers' revealed how genuine their attitudes were by initially entering their least fertile fields into the scheme for financial reasons, rather than environmental.

More organic than conventional farmers carried out conservation work, with a much higher proportion involved in the recreation of ponds, woods and hedges. This type of habitat creation is important in helping to restore agricultural sustainability to pre intensification levels. In contrast, conventional farmers saw the creation of woods and pheasant cover as conservation works. The periodicals read by the organic respondents were mainly concerned with environmental and sustainability issues other than agriculture, thereby providing insights into their attitudes towards environmental dimensions of agricultural sustainability. Membership of environmental institutions was quite low among both groups of farmers. Differences did emerge, however, reflecting attitudes towards conservation work and agricultural sustainability. Thus, while organic farmers preferred the Wildlife Trust, Woodland Trust and Friends of the Earth, conventional farmers, whose main countryside leisure pursuit is shooting, were more in favour of the Game Conservancy Trust. This supports the earlier finding that many conventional farmers see the creation of woods and pheasant cover as conservation work further suggesting that all environmental institutions are not equally 'green'.

Respondents' attitudes towards global climate change varied significantly as exemplified by more organic, than conventional farmers, environmental concern for the loss of some of the UK's most fertile agricultural land in East Anglia thereby adversely affecting agricultural sustainability. Organic farmers used this land loss as evidence of global climate change taking place due to the burning of fossil fuels. This contrasted with a number of conventional farmers who thought that such weather changes are part of the normal course of events. The attitudes of the two farmer groups were quite similar regarding the reduction of water supplies, essential for the sustainability of both types of farming, possibly because it may directly affect their livelihood.

Conventional farmers were not generally critical of GM technology and the associated potential dangers of cross-pollination of GM crops with native plant species. This contrasted with the strong ecocentric attitudes of the organic respondents who condemned GM crops totally with their perceived environmental dangers. The main reason that conventional farmers gave for not being critical of GM crops was their belief that environmental benefits would be gained from reductions in pesticide use. These findings may be related to conventional farmers anticipating future benefit from GM technology. In contrast, organic farmers may see such technology to be damaging to themselves, their families and the environment without the possibility of future benefit (Hall & Moran, 2006).

Interestingly, both groups of respondents' attitudes towards government policy regarding environmental issues such as agricultural sustainability varied considerably. On the one hand, most organic farmers believed that government policy had caused a lot of damage to the countryside and had little faith in government policy restoring such damage thus reflecting their ecocentric attitudes. On the other hand, most conventional farmers had some faith in government policy in restoring countryside damage, which they claimed was minimal thereby demonstrating their belief in the importance of a conventionally farmed countryside. However, there is a strong causal relationship between the intensification of agriculture, caused by the Common Agricultural Policy since its inception, and the decline in agricultural sustainability. For example, 620,000 miles of hedgerows were destroyed between 1984 and 1990. Such practices resulted in an average decline in farmland bird populations of 43 per cent between 1970 and 2009.

Probably somewhat unsurprisingly, the attitudes of both farmer groups varied considerably towards conventional agriculture. For example, fewer conventional than organic farmers believed that conventional agriculture has negative environmental impacts. In contrast, most organic farmers said that conventional agriculture is unsustainable because conventional farmers tend to use high levels of nitrate and pesticides on their crops. Most organic farmers were also very critical of the way in which conventional agriculture harms water quality, through pesticides usage, leading to damage to agricultural sustainability. This contrasted with conventional farmers, who believe that it is essential for them to use pesticides to grow their crops, but claimed to be aware of the dangers of over-use of such chemicals.

The attitudes of both groups of farmers towards organic farming were equally diverse, demonstrated by half of the organic respondents claiming that environmental concerns were their main reason for adopting organic methods. Significantly, half of those who emphasised environmental reasons had a degree or higher degree, possibly suggesting a link between higher education and environmental awareness. This finding is supported by Dunlap et al., (2000) who found that environmental concern was correlated with variables such as age and education. Most organic farmers said that they believed that organic agriculture is environmentally sustainable. In contrast, conventional farmers were generally not in support of those views, sometimes suggesting that organic grass farmers cause more problems with nitrates than they do, for example, by ploughing clover into their soil. Most of the organic respondents accepted that a lot of fossil fuels are used in their mechanical weeding processes. Such practices contribute to climate warming and are therefore liable to have a detrimental effect on long-term agricultural sustainability through reduced crop yield and/or failure. This suggests that organic farming systems are not always as environmentally sustainable as is often claimed.

Organic farmers' attitudes towards lowland farmland bird populations were revealed by their greater interest, knowledge and understanding of farmland avifauna than the conventional respondents. For example, some organic respondents claimed that organic farming systems are 'better' for birds than conventional agriculture. However, some conventional farmers, whilst acknowledging that intensive farming has been harmful to birds in the past, justified their opinion by blaming government agri-environmental policy for forcing them out of mixed farming. Most members of both groups of respondents had little faith in government agri-environmental policy as it relates to farmland bird populations. Many respondents were generally cynical about the government and believe they will be unsuccessful in achieving their objective of restoring farmland bird populations to 1970 levels by 2020. Importantly, Defra announced on 24th May 2012 its plans to spend £375,000 on a licensed three-year trial of Common Buzzard *Buteo buteo* capture and nest destruction on three shooting estates in Northumberland (Pitches, 2012). In contrast, possibly because of the outrage from conservationists regarding this proposal, Defra announced during the first week in July 2012 that farmers can apply for payment through agri-environmental schemes to provide supplementary food for farmland birds during their leanest months. Such mixed messages leave in considerable doubt that the government is serious in their aim of reversing the long-term declines of farmland birds and restoring sustainable populations to 1970 levels by 2020.

Generally the attitudes and behaviours revealed by the contextual life histories and work routines supported the findings revealed from the earlier analysis. For example, conventional farmers often see the creation of pheasant cover as conservation works contrasting with the more environmentally friendly attitudes of the organic farmers who often plant hedges and excavate ponds thereby helping to restore agricultural sustainability. Organic farmers' work routine was found to be more complex than the conventional respondents due to the diversity of their enterprises, thereby further contributing to farm biodiversity and agricultural sustainability.

The wide ranging differences of opinion and behaviours demonstrated by the respondents in this chapter may influence their environmental attitudes towards agricultural sustainability. It is important that the technocentric attitudes of many conventional farmers become more in line with the ecocentric attitudes of most organic farmers if long-term agricultural sustainability is to be realised. For example, similar to organic farmers, more conventional farmers could be encouraged to join agri-environmental schemes and environmental institutions with the aim of luring them from their perceived key traditional role of producers of good healthy food.

The behavioural approach adopted in this chapter proved useful in contributing towards sensitive understandings of organic and conventional farmers' perceptions, attitudes and behaviours. This was not accomplished without problems concerning the discrepancies experienced between respondents' attitudes and their physical on-farm behaviours. This study provided a conceptual and empirical contribution towards geographical research, knowledge and understandings of the environmental dimensions of agricultural sustainability in the UK.

Acknowledgements

This study could not have been carried out without the collaboration of the twenty five organic farmers and twenty five conventional farmers who took part in the 'extensive' telephone interviews. We are particularly grateful for the dedication, interest and insights provided by the five geographically linked pairs of organic and conventional farmers who generously gave of their time and shared their knowledge in the analysis of contextual life histories and work routines.

Author details

David Kings[1] and Brian Ilbery[2]

1 The Abbey, Warwick Road, Southam, Warwickshire, UK

2 Countryside and Community Research Institute, University of Gloucestershire, Oxstalls Campus, Oxstalls Lane, Longlevens, Gloucester, UK

References

[1] Alleyne, R. (2012) Storms make for the wettest start to summer in a century. *The Daily Telegraph,* 30th June 2012 p. 11.

[2] Anonymous (1999) *A Better Quality of Life – a Strategy for Sustainable Development for the United Kingdom*. DETR, London.

[3] Beedell, J. D. C. & Rehman, T. (1999) Explaining farmers' conservation behaviour: Why do farmers behave the way they do? *Journal of Environmental Management,* Vol. 57, pp. 165-176.

[4] Beedell, J. D. C. & Rehman, T. (2000) Using social-psychology models to understand farmers' conservation behaviour. *Journal of Rural Studies,* Vol. 16, pp. 117-127.

[5] Brookfield, H. C. (1969) On the environment as perceived. *Progress in Geography,* Vol. 1, pp. 51-80.

[6] Brotherton, I. (1990) Initial participation in UK Set-Aside and ESA schemes. *Planning Outlook,* Vol. 33, pp. 46-61.

[7] Buck, D., Getz, C. & Guthman, J. (1997) From farm to table: the organic vegetable commodity chain of northern California. *Sociologia Ruralis,* Vol. 37, pp. 3-19.

[8] Burn, A. J. (2000) Pesticides and their effect on lowland farmland birds. In Aebischer, N.J., Evans, A. D., Grice, P. V. & Vickery, J. A. (eds) *Ecology and Conservation of Low-land Farmland birds.* British Ornithologists' Union, Tring, pp. 89-104.

[9] Burton, R. J. F. (2004) Reconceptualising the 'Behavioural' approach in agricultural studies: a sociopsychological perspective. *Journal of Rural Studies,* Vol. 20, pp. 359-371.

[10] Cloke, P., Philo, C. & Sadler, D. (1991) *Approaching Human Geography - An Introduction to Contemporary Theoretical Debates.* Paul Chapman, London.

[11] Codex Alimentarius Commission. (1999). *What is organic agriculture?* (FAO/WHO Codex Alimentarius Commission, 1999).

[12] Coombes, B. & Campbell, H. (1998) Dependent reproduction of alternative modes of agriculture: organic farming in New Zealand. *Sociologia Ruralis,* Vol. 38, pp. 127- 145.

[13] Darnhofer, I. (2005) Organic Farming and Rural Development: Some Evidence from Austria. *Sociologia Ruralis,* Vol. 45, pp. 308-323.

[14] Defra (2002) *Countryside Stewardship Scheme* (CSS), Department for Environment, Food and Rural Affairs, London.

[15] Defra (2006) *Sustainable Farming and Food Strategy: Forward Look,* Department for Environment, Food and Rural Affairs, London.

[16] Defra (2012) *Farmers are to be paid for feeding farmland birds,* Department for Environment, Food and Rural Affairs, London.

[17] Dunlap, R. E., Van Liere, K. D., Mertig, A. G. & Jones, R. E. (2000) Measuring endorsement of the New Ecological Paradigm: a revised NEP scale. *Journal of Social Issues,* Vol. 56, pp. 425-442.

[18] Edward-Jones, G. & Howells, O. (2001) The origin and hazard of inputs to crop protection in organic farming systems: are they sustainable? *Agricultural Systems,* Vol. 67, pp. 31- 47.

[19] Farshad, A. & Zinck. J. A. (2003) Seeking agricultural sustainability. *Agriculture, Ecosystems and Environment,* Vol. 47, pp. 1-12.

[20] Fuller, R. J. (1997) Responses of birds to organic arable farming: mechanisms and evidence. *Proceedings 1997 Brighton Crop Protection Conference - Weeds.* British Crop Protection Council, Farnham, pp. 897-906.

[21] Gasson, R. (1974) Socio-economic status and orientation to work: the case of farmers. *Sociologia Ruralis,* Vol. 14, pp. 127-141.

[22] Gillmor, D. (1986) Behavioural studies in agriculture: goals, values and enterprise choice. *Irish Journal of Agricultural Economics and Rural Sociology,* Vol. 11, pp. 19-33.

[23] Godfray, C. J., Crute, I., Haddad, L., Lawrence, D., Muir, J. F., Nisbett, N., Pretty, J., Robinson, S., Toulmin, C. & Whiteley, R. (2010) The future of the global food system. *Phil. Trans. R. Soc. B,* Vol. 365, pp. 2769-2777.

[24] Gray, L. (2012) Embrace GM 'if you want cheap food.' *The Daily Telegraph,* 1st June 2012.

[25] Guthman, J. (2004) The Trouble with 'Organic Lite' in California: a Rejoiner to the 'Conventionalisation' Debate. *Sociologia Ruralis,* Vol. 44, pp. 301-316.

[26] Hall, J. (2012a) Worst drought since 1976. *The Daily Telegraph,* 16th April 2012.

[27] Hall, J. (2012b) Wettest April ends drought in 19 counties. *The Daily Telegraph,* 12th May 2012.

[28] Hall, A. & Mogyorody, V. (2001) Organic farmers in Ontario: an examination of the conventionalisation argument. *Sociologia Ruralis,* Vol. 41, pp. 399-422.

[29] Hall, C. & Moran, D. (2006) Investigating GM risk perceptions: A survey of anti-GM and environmental campaign group members. *Journal of Rural Studies,* Vol. 22, pp. 29- 37.

[30] Hansen, B., Alroe, H. F. & Kristensen, E. (2001) Approaches to assess the environmental impact of organic farming with particular regard to Denmark. *Agriculture, Ecosystems and Environment,* Vol. 55, pp. 11-26.

[31] Ilbery, B. W. (1978) Agricultural decision-making: a behavioural perspective. *Progress in Human Geography,* Vol. 2, pp. 448-466.

[32] Ilbery, B. W. (1985) Factors affecting the structure of horticulture in the Vale of Evesham, UK: a behavioural interpretation. *Journal of Rural Studies,* Vol. 1, pp. 121-133.

[33] Ilbery, B. W., Holloway, L., & Arber, R. (1999) The geography of organic farming in England and Wales in the 1990s. *Tijdschrift voor Economische en Sociale Geografie,* Vol. 90, pp. 285-295.

[34] Ilbery, B. & Maye, D. (2005) Food supply chains and sustainability: evidence from specialist food producers in the Scottish/English borders. *Land Use Policy,* Vol. 22, pp. 331- 344.

[35] International Federation of Organic Agriculture Movements (2008) Press release 22nd January 2010.

[36] Kings, D. & Ilbery, B. (2010) The environmental belief systems of organic and conventional farmers: Evidence from central-southern England. *Journal of Rural Studies,* Vol. 26, 437-448.

[37] Kings, D. & Ilbery, B. (2011) Farmers' Attitudes Towards Organic and Conventional Agriculture: A Behavioural Perspective. In: Reed, M. (ed) *Organic Food and Agriculture: New Trends and Developments in the Social Sciences.* InTech, Open Access Publishers, pp. 145-168.

[38] Lampkin, N. (1990) *Organic Farming.* Farming Press, Ipswich.

[39] Lang, T. & Barling, D. (2012) (forthcoming) Food Security or Food Sustainability: The return and reformulation of an old debate. *Geographical Journal.*

[40] Lockie, S. & Halpin, D. (2005) The Conventionalisation thesis reconsidered: structural and idealogical transformation of Australian organic agriculture. *Sociologia Ruralis,* Vol. 45, pp. 284-307.

[41] Lotter, D. (2003) Organic agriculture. *Journal of Sustainable Agriculture,* Vol. 21, pp. 59-128.

[42] Maye, D. & Ilbery, B. (2011) Changing geographies of food production. In: Daniels, P., Sidaway, J., Shaw, D. & Bradshaw, M. (eds) *Introduction to human geography*. Pearson Educational, Harlow.

[43] Maxey, L. (2007) From 'Alternative' to 'Sustainable' Food. In Maye, D., Holloway, L. & Kneafsey, M. (Eds) *Alternative Food Geographies: Concepts and Debates.* Elsevier, Oxford.

[44] Mellanby, K. (1967) *Pesticides and Pollution.* Collins, London.

[45] Mellanby, K. (1970) *Environmental Pollution*. Applied Science Publishers Ltd, London.

[46] Mellanby, K. (1981) *Farming and Wildlife*. Collins, London.

[47] Moore, N. W. (1962) Toxic chemicals and birds: the ecological background to conservation problems. *British Birds,* Vol. 55, pp. 428-436.

[48] Moore, N. W. (1966) (ed) Pesticides in the Environment and their Effects on Wild Life. The Proceedings of a NATO Advanced Study Institute sponsored by the North Atlantic Treaty Organization. Monks Wood Experimental Station. *Journal of Applied Ecology,* Vol. 3, Suplement.

[49] Moore, N. W. (1970) Pesticides know no frontiers. *New Scientist*, Vol. 46, pp. 114-115.

[50] Moore, N. W. & Ratcliffe, D. A. (1962) Chlorinated residues in the eggs of a Peregrine Falcon (*Falco peregrinus*) from Perthshire. *Bird Study*, Vol. 9, pp. 242-244.

[51] Moore, N. W. & Walker, C. H. (1964) Organic chloride insecticide residues in wild birds. *Nature*, Vol. 201, pp. 1072-1073.

[52] Morgan, K. & Murdoch, J. (2000) Organic vs. conventional agriculture: knowledge, power and innovation in the food chain. *Geoforum,* Vol. 13, pp. 159-173.

[53] Morris, C. & Potter, C. (1995) Recruiting the new conservationists: farmers' adoption of agri- environmental schemes in the UK. *Journal of Rural Studies,* Vol. 11, pp. 51-63.

[54] O'Riordan, T. (1981) *Environmentalism* (second edition). Pion, London.

[55] O'Riordan, T. (1997) *Ecotaxation and the sustainability transition*. In: O'Riordan, T. (ed) Ecotaxation. Earthscan, London, pp. 7-20.

[56] Pitches, A. (2012) Defra cancels plan for state-sanctioned Buzzard persecution. *British Birds*, Vol. 105, pp. 424-425.

[57] Plimer, I. (2009) *Heaven and Earth – Global Warming: The Missing Science*. Quartet Books, London.

[58] Pugliese, P. (2001) Organic farming and sustainable rural development: a multifaceted and promising convergence. *Sociologia Ruralis,* Vol. 41, pp. 112-130.

[59] Ratcliffe, D. A. (1962) Breeding density in the Peregrine *Falco peregrinus* and Raven *Corvus corax*. *Ibis*, Vol. 104, pp. 13-39.

[60] Ratcliffe, D. A. (1963) The status of the Peregrine in Great Britain 1963-64. *Bird Study*, Vol. 10, pp. 56-90.

[61] Redclift, M. (1987) *Sustainable development: exploring the contradictions*. Methuen, London.

[62] Redclift, M. (1992) The meaning of sustainable development. *Geoforum*, Vol. 23, pp. 395-403.

[63] Rosin, C. & Campbell, H. (2009) 'Beyond bifurcation: examining the conventions of organic agriculture in New Zealand'. *Journal of Rural Studies*, Vol. 25, pp. 35-47.

[64] Shoard, M. (1980) *The theft of the countryside*. Temple-Smith, London.

[65] Sotherton, N. W. & Self, M. J. (2000) Changes in plant and arthropod biodiversity on lowland farms: an overview. In: Aebischer, N.J., Evans, A. D., Grice, P. V. & Vickery, J. A. (eds) *Ecology and Conservation of Lowland Farmland birds*. British Ornithologists' Union, Tring, pp. 105-114.

[66] RSPB (2011) *Wind farms*. Locational Guidance Publications.

[67] Storkey, J., Meyer, S., Still, K. S. & Leuschner, C. (2011) The impact of agricultural intensification and land-use on the European arable flora. *Proc. R. Soc. B rspb20111686.*

[68] Willer, H. & Gillmor, D. (1992) Organic Farming in the Republic of Ireland. *Irish Geography*, Vol. 25, pp. 149-159.

[69] Wilson, G. A. (1996) Farmer environmental attitudes and ESA participation. *Geoforum*, Vol. 27, pp. 115-131.

[70] Wilson, G. A. (1997) Factors influencing farmer participation in the Environmentally Sensitive Areas scheme. *Journal of Environmental Management*, Vol. 50, pp. 67-93.

[71] Wood,W. (2000) Attitude change; persuasion and influence. *Annual Review of Psychology*, Vol. 51, pp. 539-570.

[72] Wolpert, J. (1964) The decision process in spatial context. *Annals of the Association of American Geographers*, Vol. 5, pp. 537-538.

[73] World Commission on Environment and development (1987) *Our common future*. Oxford University Press, Oxford.

Chapter 7

Production and Distribution of Organic Foods: Assessing the Added Values

Leila Hamzaoui-Essoussi and Mehdi Zahaf

Additional information is available at the end of the chapter

http://dx.doi.org/10.5772/52445

1. Introduction

Looking at the present food chain, concerns are related to anxiety among consumers about the quality of the food they eat, GMOs, use of pesticides and antibiotics, and industrialization of the agricultural system. Growing consumer demand for organic food (OF) is based on most of these facts [1, 2]. Although OF is generally considered to present less risk than conventional foods, this debate has been re-launched as a direct consequence of rising concerns related to risks associated with intensive agricultural production, food industrialization, and the effects of food technologies and food scares [1, 3]. An increasing number of organic brands, certification labels, and wider range of organic product categories has been observed in terms of efforts to provide higher food safety and food quality. But these factors do not seem to have increased consumers' perceived value of organic food products nor trust in OF. Moreover, consumers seem to be ambivalent about channels of distribution as trust/mistrust appears to be an important factor in deciding, not only where to buy products, but also whether to buy OF products or not [17].

From the production and supply side, there are some unique challenges to the cost and logistics of moving locally or regionally produced organic food to the market. Of particular interest are the operations size and the situation of small and medium size farms. The production of the latter is of little interest to mainstream grocery chains as it is limited to a few hundred tons. Among other factors, production methods and operations size are key here. Large-scale farming is sustained by important economies of scale while small scale farming leads to higher prices. This covers the extra costs of not using fertilizers and antibiotics. As a result, there is a wide variety of product classifications depending on the production methods and thus, the operations' size. This in turn gives raise to 2 distinct distribution systems: long channels, eg. retail chains, that add value through price and high distribution intensity, and short channels, eg. direct from producers, that add value through their production methods and sustainable practices. Hence, discrepancies between market realities, the value chain and the value delivery system are still a challenge for the organic food sector. The main issue here is to determine the factors on which the different production methods and distribution systems rely on in order to add value to the organic food products offered. This study first presents the current literature related to the structure of the production and distribution of the organic food system and market, supported by an integrative production-distribution model. The model integrates the different levels of the production/supply side key factors. Challenges and strategies that add value to the organic food products are analyzed. These strategies are used by (i) the pre-supply, (ii) the supply/production, and (iii) the distribution channels.

2. The organic food system

2.1. Organic food product classification

From a production standpoint, there are various categories of production methods. In Canada, there are three main classes of production labels: (i) organic, (ii) transitional organic, and (iii) all other labels regrouping local, natural, pesticide-free and ecologically friendly. The first product class is well defined and regulated since 2009, while the second and third categories are neither - clearly - defined nor regulated.

The use of the term "organic" is restricted to farms, products, processors and other intermediaries in the value chain between production and consumption which has been certified by Certifying Bodies (CB). These CBs are independent and private fee-for-service agencies that are generally overseen by National Food Inspection Agencies. Organic certification is an arduous process which, if enacted on a farm previously farmed using conventional methods, requires at least three years to ensure all chemicals have leached from the soil and that organic amendments have had the opportunity to rebuild soil fertility.

"Transitional organic" is also a restricted label and describes farms which have made the commitment to move toward organic certification. For instance, the "transitional" label is applied to farms label is applied, for example, to farms which have switched to certifiable organic methods and are in the 36-month period between the last use of chemicals and the time the land can be assumed free of chemicals, and the farm can be certified organic.

Labels like "local", "natural", "pesticide-free" and "ecologically friendly" are not regulated and tend to be used by small farms catering to local/regional clientele. With the exception of marketing board-regulated products like dairy or chicken, production and handling of foods sold under these labels is for the most part not monitored or regulated except by governmental agencies and district health units. As a result information on farms operating outside of the organic certification system is scattered and incomplete.

Lastly, "organic" foods have to be differentiated from "functional" foods [4]. Organic foods tend to be regulated and are based on supply side value while functional foods are not very regulated and are based on demand side value. While both types of product are marketed to achieve the same objective, i. e. healthy products, the market positioning is very different.

2.2. Organic food production

According to the Canadian General Standards Board, "Organic production is a holistic system designed to optimize the productivity and fitness of diverse communities within the agro-ecosystem, including soil organisms, plants, livestock and people. The principal goal of organic production is to develop enterprises that are sustainable and harmonious with the environment. " [5]. It is worth noting that the organic movement, which began as an alternative style of production among small farms looking both to reduce their environmental footprint and to differentiate their products from commercially produced foods, has been admitted to the mainstream market. Certification, which came about to prevent fraudulent claims, has enabled large players to get into the game, facilitating the long-distance shipping and distribution of organic products required to bring them to grocery stores and wholesale clubs. It applies within the value chain the same downward pressure on price exhibited in the conventional food value chain. This has resulted, for some small farmers concerned with the philosophical aspects of organic production, in diminished credibility of the organic standard and a refusal to participate. It has also hardened the value chain against entry by these small farmers [6].

Further, to be qualified as organic, processed foods must be processed in certified facilities. Added-value processing in Canada is limited by the small number of certified processors. Handlers of organic products must also be certified. This is the other major factor, and one that could mitigate the seasonality of foods: further processing could provide a wider market and a longer selling window for perishables. By characterizing producers' use of the value chain to get products to the consumer, we can break the organic producers down into three categories: large, small and medium-sized operations.

Large producers are characterized by organic cash crops, which are either exported or processed after they leave the farm, by livestock or field crops which are most likely to go to distributors and processors for further treatment [7]. Most dairy farms would be considered large producers in this context.

Medium-sized producers tend to produce for a smaller geographical market [7]. Limited by infrastructure, some of these producers are now working together to develop their own products, partnering up with complementary businesses to be able to expand the offerings of their on-farm market to attract more customers. Others have partnered with small regional processor/distributors to reach restaurants and specialty food retailers. Most medium producers offer on-farm markets as stationary storefronts, incorporating products sold on consignment or retailed for other area producers.

Small organic producers tend to not use distribution intermediaries. Instead they focus on direct relationships with consumers through farmers' markets and on-farm markets. They may supply some restaurants, specialty retailers, or small grocers, but these relationships are painstakingly developed and rely on niche marketing and personal relationships. These are the small farms most likely to give up on organic certification due to the paperwork and expenses involved.

2.3. Organic food distribution

In conventional food systems, there exists between producers and consumers of food products a series of handlers involved in the processing and distribution. Since organic products have entered into the mainstream market, a similar mainstream value chain has developed for organic products being sold through conventional outlets. Traditional retail, with its focus on profit, seeks consistent supplies of products. Imports from warmer climates offer this consistency; we see California and Mexico lettuce occupying shelves year-round because, for reasons of efficiency, retailers prefer to deal with a single supplier rather than displace the year-round supplier with a seasonally-available product.

Organic food has emerged as an important segment of food retailing in recent years. The organic food industry has steadily moved from niche markets, e. g. , small specialty stores, to mainstream markets, e. g. , large supermarket chains [8, 9]. Ten years ago the bulk of OF sales were made in specialty stores (95%) while the remaining 5% were realized in mainstream stores. Nowadays, the trend has been reversed [10]. Farmers' markets among other alternative distribution channels are being used and are characterized by a direct link between the producer and the consumer [11]. In some countries, distributors are promoting their own line of OF products under specific brand names [12, 13, 14].

In Canada, the total annual retail sales of certified organic products in 2009 were approximately $2 billion, with about 45% moving through mainstream supermarkets [15], and OF retail sales represented 1% of total retail food sales. More specifically, total mass market sales of certified OF products approximated CA $586 million allocated as follow: CA $175 million through small grocery stores, drug stores, and specialty stores, and CA $411 million in large grocery chains. These figures do not account for alternative distribution channels such as farmers' markets, natural food stores, box delivery, and other channels such as restaurants. These channels totalize CA $415 million [16]. Conventional distribution channels, characterized by a longer channel where consumers do not see and interact with the producer and where the information about food is limited, is targeted toward consumers that look for a one-stop grocery shopping experience [6, 17]. These are the regular OF consumers. On the other hand, channels such as box delivery, specialty stores, and small grocery stores or even direct channels such as the farmer's market are targeted toward consumers that look to interact – socially - with the producers [11], ask them questions about their production methods, food origin and variety, and cooking tips. These are the hardcore consumers. Most of the demand is coming from Europe and North America and these two regions are not self-sufficient. The main problem for producers and growers is to supply this demand. Large volumes of organic imports, coming in from other regions, are used to balance the undersupply. US sales of organic products grew in 2009 by 5. 3%, to reach 26. 6 billion US dollars, representing 3. 7% of the food market. In Europe, sales of organic products approximated EU 18'400 million in 2009 [18]. The largest market for organic products in

2009 was Germany (5. 8 billion euros) followed by France (3 billion euros) and the UK (2 billion euros).

3. The organic food market

The organic food market is characterized by consumers buying organic food products for different motivations and values. OF consumers also have different buying processes that are not the result of one decision but a series of decisions nested in each other. Among these, decisions about where to buy is here considered as it directly relates to consumers' most used and trusted distribution channels.

3.1. Consumers' motivations to buy organic food products

Through the literature, several motivations to buy organic food have been identified and ranked. Personal health remains a strong motivating factor, organic food products being perceived as less associated with health risk than conventional food products [19]. Concerns for the environment and for animals' wellbeing appear as other reasons for buying organic food [20, 21, 22]. Issues about food quality but also "eating to enjoy" is mentioned to be important motivations for OF consumption in several countries like France, Italy and Greece [23, 24]. Furthermore, tasty and nourishing products are considered as important motivations and [25] found that most organic consumers think that organic food tastes better than conventional. Last, organic products are associated by fewer consumers with local production because they like to support the local economy [6, 26]. The cultural differences cause consumers in different countries to have various motivations with regard to OF, such as health and tradition in France vs. health and environment in Sweden [2, 27].

In their study, [29] provided an overview of the personal motivations of organic food consumption within a framework linking these motivations to Schwartz' values theory. When considering health as a motivation for purchasing organic food, it appears that consumers link it with the value of security, or safety and harmony. Good taste and eating to enjoy relates to hedonism or pleasure and sensuous gratification for oneself. The propensity to behave in an environment-friendly way (environment and animal welfare) relates to the value of universalism whereas supporting the local economy is related to the value of benevolence. But this latter is only highlighted in fewer studies. This is even more interesting as an important share of organic food is still imported because OF markets are not self-sufficient.

3.2. Trust in the organic foods distribution system

Given the prevailing climate of food-related fear and consumer uncertainty, trust indicators may have a significant role to play. Perceived risks pertaining to food consumption and lack of knowledge regarding organic products are leading consumers to rely on different indicators such as brand name, store image, label or partners like producers. Consumers' trust toward the distribution channels also appear to be an important factor in deciding not only where to buy but also what to buy. This highlights the importance of examining the trust issue from the supply side. Indeed, the main OF market actors are contributing, at different levels and with different strategies to consumers' level of knowledge of, preferences for, as well as trust/mistrust in OF products. As a matter of fact, building trust in the OF supply requires tools such as quality certification or labeling that have to be established and used as a promotion strategy. Trust orientations should be studied in the context of market actors such as producers/farmers and distributors or certifying bodies. Since markets differ in how the food system is organized, each player (producers/farmers, distributors, certifiers) adds a different value to the product and requires distinct distribution flows to do so. This is very likely to be in direct relation with the type of consumers and their preferred and most used channels of distribution.

4. Objectives and framework

Whereas the majority of previous research is focusing on the demand side, this study aims to uncover variations among supply side players (producers/farmers, distributors, certifiers) with regards to the OF supply chain and factors they rely on to add value to organic products. This value needs to be determined and estimated at all levels of the channel of distribution. Further, the logistics of the value delivery network need to be investigated. This will lead to an in-depth understanding of the value added in the organic food distribution system, the current market structure, as well as the determination of the challenges faced by the major players of the organic food industry. A second objective is to identify the different distribution strategies and arrangements to market organic foods and increase trust in OF products. Building trust in the OF supply requires more than just ensuring product quality and product knowledge, labeling or setting proper pricing and communication strategies, as trust is missing at various levels of the marketing value delivery system and the food supply chain. The dimensions of trust necessary to achieve market growth have to be integrated to the OF product positioning and the distribution strategies. In their effort to rebuild consumer confidence and satisfy consumer demand, such information is important for all market participants involved in the supply food system. Lastly, to support these two objectives it is important to provide a precise and useful profile of organic food consumers in relation with their preferred channel of distribution and main trust orientations.

To address the abovementioned objectives, our approach is based on an integrative production-distribution model (cf. Figure 1). There are 3 layers of decisions in this model (i) presupply: this is related to certification decisions, laws and regulations related to government agencies, and finally expert opinions on the industry structure and evolution, (ii) supply: this is related to the production, production methods, imports, and sold quantities, and (iii) channels of distribution: broken down into 3 main categories, long or standard channel, short channels, and direct channels.

http://dx.doi.org/10. 5772/52445

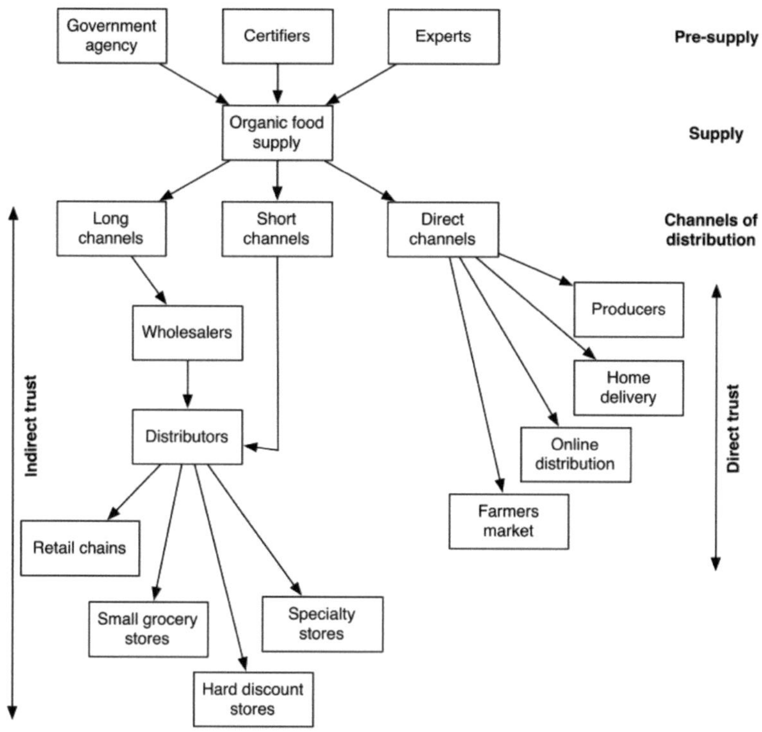

Figure 1. Integrative Production-Distribution Model

5. Design and procedure

5.1. Design

The abovementioned objectives require a 2-level design. This design determines how distributors/producers manage similarities and differences between what consumers want and what they offer them. A supply-side study has been developed to assess the production-distribution model. This in turn will lead to the development of a second model that takes also into account the demand-side (production/market model). First, in the supply-side study, secondary data on the organic food industry was collected to understand its market structure; then in-depth interviews were conducted with producers, distributors and certifiers. Distributors and producers were profiled as follow: (i) by channel size and type, (ii) by organic food products variety, and (iii) by channel position (retailer, wholesaler, etc.). Further, there is a three-prong challenge related to the interviews quality and consistency: (i) interviews had to cover a wide range of producers and distributors in the organic food industry, (ii) interviewees had to be decision makers or gate keepers in their channels of distribution/

organization, and (iii) the sample size should be sufficient enough to ensure consistency of the results without reaching any saturation.

5.2. Qualitative and quantitative procedures

Secondary data was collected in Canada using major sources of information as well as informal interviews with 14 industry key players (experts, certifiers, and government represen-taitves). As gatekeepers to the organic label, these key players can provide the most recent and accurate information about the numbers and types of organic farms, products and businesses, as private enterprises, are under no obligation to do so. Information obtained from these gatekeepers, while fairly comprehensive within its scope, is not necessarily accurate. This is illustrated by the example that, in order to reach various target export markets, some farms, products and businesses are certified by multiple bodies simultaneously. Lastly, 2 sets of in-depth interviews, based on 2 thematic interview guides that lasted about 30 minutes to 45 minutes, were conducted with 90 respondents (cf. Table 1). The first set of interviews focuses on the production/supply aspects while the second set focuses on the distribution/market, and hence the distribution logistics and its impact on the consumer's market. The interviews were recorded (digital voice recorder), transcribed, coded, and analyzed using content analysis [30]. This technique allows the researcher to include large amounts of textual information and methodically identifies its properties by detecting important structures of its content. Two separate judges coded the data to ensure a minimum of 80% correspondence.

Interviewees	Production/ distribution	Distribution/ market
Retail chains	0	7
Small grocery stores	0	2
Specialty stores	0	12
Organic producers/farmers' markets	15	17
Certifiers	0	8
Organic food experts	0	7
Other distributors	15	7
Total	30	60

Table 1. Interviews by Distributor Type

5.3. Research tools

The secondary data analysis led to the compilation of information coming from various sources, then information gaps were determined. These gaps relate to discrepancies between dollar sales and dollar production, the characterization of the value delivery system, and exports/imports of organic foods. Results from this phase have been used to design and structure both interview guides:

- The production/supply interview guide is composed of 5 sections; 3 sections related to marketing mix elements of organic foods (product, price, and place), a 4th section about the organic food market, and the last section deals with certification and labeling.
- The distribution/market interview guide is composed of three main sections. The first section probes distributors to discuss their perceptions of the current OF market and the structure of their distribution channel. The second and third sections deal with distributors' perception of consumers' concerns, trust issues related to their distribution strategies, and how consumers' concerns are addressed.

These 2 sets of interviews are complementary. Hence, the analyses have been combined for the sake of obtaining more exhaustive and integrative results. 59 keywords, clustered in 13 themes, have been generated from the interviews transcriptions. These themes are classified as follow: (i) production and supply: the section presents the challenges and issues that producers/farmers deals with when marketing their organic foods; (ii) value delivery system: value creation throughout the distribution channels; (iii) market/industry structure: this theme category covers various market trends and the demand as perceived by the supply side, (iv) distribution strategies: this section groups all distribution strategies as well as distribution logistics; (v) trust issues: these are consumers concerns regarding OF and the corresponding distribution strategies used to increase trust; and (vi) sustainability: this last category deals with the impact of sustainability on the organic food industry.

6. Findings

6.1. Production and supply

Information on the production of organic foods tends to be collected and provided in terms of acreage in production and not in final retail sales value, making it difficult to bridge between production and economic value. Retail numbers, when provided, are generally estimated based on current market values and expected yields by acre for the crops in production. They do not account for any added-value processing which may occur between the producer and the consumer. Further, because certifying bodies deal only with certified or transitional organic products and businesses, their numbers do not reflect the uncounted number of small mixed-production farms operating outside of the certification process. These farms are selling under one of the "natural" and "local" alternative labels commonly used in direct-to-customer sales at Farmers' Markets and on-farm stores.

By characterizing producers' use of the value chain to get products to the consumer, organic producers can be broken down into three categories: large, small and medium-sized operations. Like the medium-sized farming/processing operations, larger processing and distribution centers tend to co-pack with conventional products, ensuring sufficient throughout to be profitable. These enterprises tend to be closed systems; like the large retail outlets they serve, those are interested mainly in consistency of product and supply and so they contract with large growers for their raw products. Smaller packing, processing and distribution operations are often spawned by the producers themselves as a way of making their products more marketable. This adds value and extends the selling window for their own products; basically building in forward integration of the value chain. To maintain year-round clientele these operations supplement with organic imports on a seasonal basis and retail the products of other producers.

There seems to be little overlap between large, medium and small producers at the processing, distribution and sales stages. There is very little shared infrastructure between these levels. The processing and distribution system for large producers is, for the most part, closed; it's available to those large producers only. The system for the medium-sized producers, developed by those same medium-sized producers, tends to remain closed because they are still struggling to maintain their position; they've done enormous amounts of work in establishing themselves and often consider the information and infrastructure they've developed to be proprietary.

6.2. Value delivery system

It is clear from the interviews that the organic food system tends to echo the conventional system in terms of the size and distribution of margin within the value chain - more details will be given in the upcoming sections. There are effectively three distribution chains of increasing efficiency at work in the organic food system, culminating in three types of retail. As in any distribution structure, every intermediary involved in the organic value chain must be able to add sufficient margin to cover its operating costs and generate enough profit to justify continued operation. The final price paid by the consumer reflects a share paid to each participant. This price must also be low enough to be attractive to consumers. Entry into the market of large supermarket chains has had a significant impact on price, producing downward pressure on the value chain in much the same way it has occurred in the conventional chain. While this has made organics more accessible and increased the volume of sales, the return to a focus on price has decreased the value of the organic label to small farmers.

Further to this, according to the supply side, distributors perform different distribution flows, thus creating distinct "organic values" sold through their channel of distribution. The "organic value" is directly related to the efficiency of the value delivery system. It is also clear that there are two distribution perspectives: long/medium size channels such as retail chains and small grocery stores versus short channel such as specialty stores, farmers' market, and producers. Long/medium channels have a price/variety driven value, while short channels offer a value based on traceability and quality. This supports the importance of pricing. Prices tend to be higher in shorter channels than in longer channels as there are more flows performed by fewer channel members. Hence, shorter channels need larger margins to stay in business.

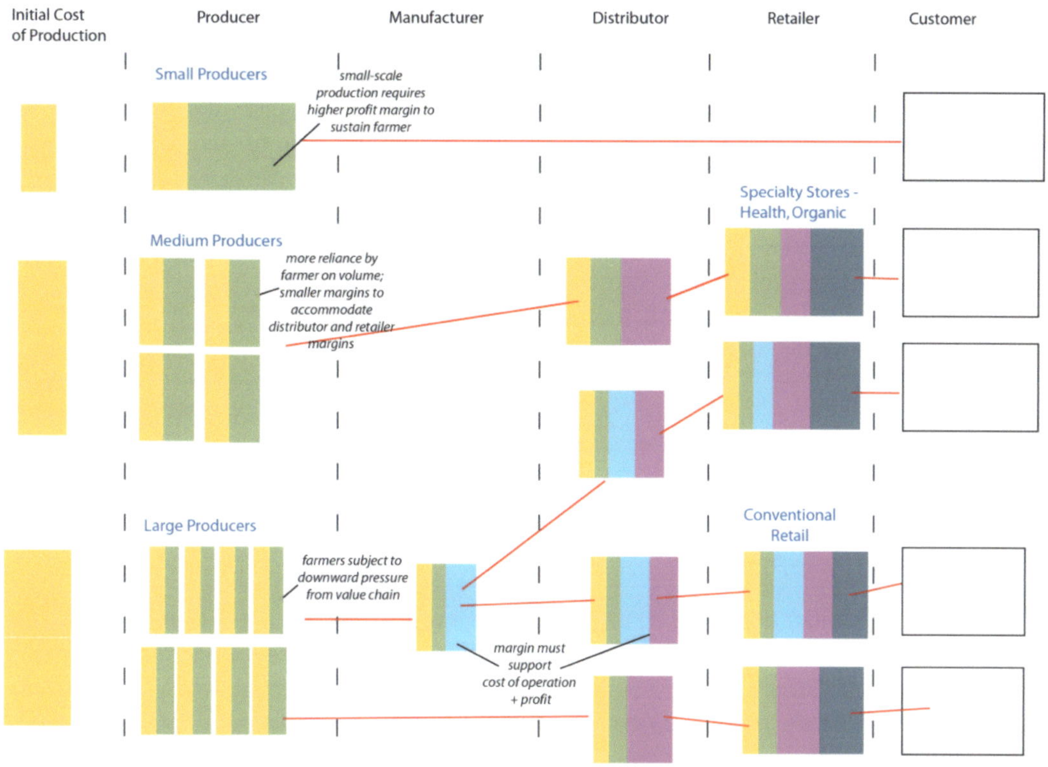

Figure 2. Organic Value Creation

6.3. Market/industry structure

In terms of product lifecycle, the OF market is not at maturity yet. Overall, distributors agree that the OF market is growing and shows substantial opportunities. More specifically they mentioned an increasing diversification of product lines and channels of distribution. Most of these distributors argued that the organic food market is demand driven; it is basically based on a derived demand, *"I am wishing, that at the retail level, we would have a better supply of it to meet the demands of our customers"*. This demand is exponentially growing, leading distributors to rely more and more on imports to compensate the under-supplied of local and national production. Further, many conventional channels are increasing their organic sales adopting conventional marketing strategies to organic food products; including organic versions of conventional brands. This is done to satisfy the needs of wider OF segments. The increasing number of distribution channels is also based on an increasing number of supermarkets and food store chains offering and widening their offer of organic foods at very competitive prices. Further, with the growth in popularity of organic food products, many wholesalers have entered the organic food supply chain. They have been encouraged by chain stores that need larger quantities at regular delivery times, and have to work through them because of high demand, *"I am wishing, that at the retail level, we would have a better supply of it to meet the demands of our customers"*. Consequently, imports from regions with large organic farming activities (eg. California) still prevails. The second major trend is pricing. All interviewees including distributors, certifiers, and experts agree that price is a key factor to enhance organic foods demand. However, price has been more discussed as a cost-control tool rather then as a market price-sensitivity issue, *"but one of the most difficult things is to make it price competitive"*. It is clear that the industry is slowly moving toward a price skimming strategy. Third, all interviewees agree to say that consumers are becoming more educated and make smarter food choices. However, there are clear differences in their purchasing behavior. Producers and farmers' markets managers stated that their customers have specific needs and motivations to buy organic foods, such as health and support of local farmers. Conversely, consumers buying from conventional channels, i. e. retail chains, are looking for a different shopping and consumption experience. This is directly related to the OF adoption process. Consumers trusting the labels and certifications are in the interest-evaluation-trial phase while consumers trusting stores are in the adoption phase.

6.4. Distribution strategies

The increasing number of distribution channels seems to be mainly based on an increasing number of supermarkets and food store chains offering OF products and widening their offer of organic foods at more competitive prices. As a matter of fact, the diversification of the offer is the main driver of the market growth for supermarkets and retail chain managers. Most conventional channels are increasing their organic sales using conventional marketing strategies for organic food (like offering organic versions of conventional brands). This helps satisfying the needs of a wider number of OF segments.

From the producers and farmers' perspective, being able to expand supply is a big issue that translates into poor supply reliability and poor availability at the demand level. More wholesalers have entered the organic food supply chain with the growth in popularity of organic food products. They have been encouraged by chain stores because demand is up and they need larger quantities at regular delivery times, and wholesalers are key here. Consequently, imports from other regions with large organic farming activities still prevails. On the other hand, "local food" consumption is starting to drive the organic food demand. These products are a superior quality alternative to what is called "industrial organic" offered in supermarkets and retail chains. Producers are also making efforts in diversifying their offering and widening their product lines. It is interesting to note that direct channels offer competitive prices with regards to retail chain and supermarket. This represents a serious alternative for consumers looking to buy organic.

From the organic food specialty stores' perspective (independent stores as well as small chain stores), the organic market shows differences with supermarkets in terms of variety, price and quality. In other words, supermarkets are able to provide consumers with a larger variety, lower prices and convenience whereas specialty stores differentiate themselves with the quality and the origin of their products. The main difference between suppliers is determined in terms of short-direct/long channel of distribution, with producers offering traceability and quality. This is also related to the value offered in these channels: price versus quality.

6.5. Trust issues and distribution

6.5.1. Trust issues

Consumers have different trust orientations/levels depending on the type of distribution channel they use: trust related to labeling and certification, trust in the store selling OF, and trust in the production origin. Table 2 presents the distributors perspective on consumers' trust and ways to increase trust in organic food products.

Distributors	Trust more	Trust less	To Increase trust
Retail chains	Product labels ++ Certification labels +	Brands	Price Accuracy Consumers' education Quality
Small Grocery Stores	Product labels ++ Store reputation ++ Store manager ++	Brands	Consumer education Knowing the producer Price accuracy
Specialty stores	Product labels ++ Certification labels ++	Brands	Consumers' education Quality
			Consumers' education Knowing the producer
Organic producers	Certification labels + Production methods ++	NA	Consumers' education
Certifiers/ Experts	Certification labels ++	NA	Information on the labels Consumers' education Knowing the producer Production methods Certification process
Other distributors	Product labels ++ Certification labels +	NA	

Table 2. Trust Levels by Distributors

Retail chain managers mention – unanimously – that the product label is important. They also acknowledge that there are different types of consumers based on their level of trust. Consumers buying in these outlets feel very confortable knowing what to buy and finding all information they look for. Retail chains selling organics use intensive distribution strategies, as their customers are also looking for a one-stop shopping experience. Hence, convenience and price are the main drives of the organic value here. This relegates other product attributes such as certification, brand name and country of origin to a passive role. From a strategic standpoint, retail chain managers are using conventional marketing strategies to increase their OF market share. For instance, price-skimming strategies, shelf-space and shelf life, as well as product differentiation are used to penetrate this fast growing market segment. Conversely, the organic value marketed in small grocery stores is mainly based on the relationship with the manager, the store reputation and also on the product/certification label. Managers' strategies are mainly targeted towards store loyalty; consumers trust the store hence they trust the manager, *"I would guess trust because the consumer is trusting me as a store owner"*. Since the clientele base is smaller than in chain stores, managers are more approachable and they know some of their customers by name. This enhances the trust relationship between the store and the consumers, which is very important to stay afloat and in business. Further, this is a guarantee for quality and counterbalances the lack of brand effect. Lastly, managers argue that consumers buying in their store are knowledgeable and ask about specific product attributes when buying organic. As for retail chains, branding is not important.

Specialty stores managers observe that consumers trust labels, i. e. , product label and certification label. The value offered in this channel is based on the width and depth of the product lines, and also on the traceability of organic foods via certification labels. Hence, labeling is important as a source of information. Managers acknowledge also that OF consumers are more knowledgeable; thus they are able to recognize and also to evaluate the different certification labels. What is interesting though is that managers do not see any difference between consumers with regards to their trust level. It is important to note that even if brands are crucial to position the store offering, brands are not used to increase trust in this market.

Most organic producers and farmers' markets managers acknowledged that consumers trust certification. This is important, especially knowing that not all producers are certified. They say that when consumers approach them to buy organic foods, they look for certification labels. However, when producers discuss the production methods with them, when they show them around, consumers start building a trust relationship that acts as a certification seal, *"I think that's part of the trust, to open your farm and have it open for your customers so they can come and see"*. Therefore, the organic value is based on the production methods. This value offsets price sensitivity and the need for branding.

Lastly, other distributors, such as wholesalers, reiterate the importance of labeling and pricing, but they also add a new emerging and fast growing trend: local foods. The discussion revolved around several aspects of "local foods". Some relate it to organics saying that there is a clear difference between what they called "industrial organic" – sold through long channels – and "local organic" – sold through short channels. Furthermore, some said that more consumers want to buy local even if it is not organic, *"the fact that the product is organic is less important than the fact that it is direct selling"*. This, obviously, deepens the divide between the market segments.

To recapitulate, there are several market clusters based on distinct trust orientations and distinct organic values. Consumers rely on various cues to build their trust in the OF products offered in all distribution channels. Labeling – product labeling and certification labeling - plays a key role to inform consumers and strengthen trust whereas brands do not add to the level of trust in OF whatever the type of distribution channel. Last, local foods and local organic foods represent serious new trends in the industry. Trust orientations depend also on the channel length. Long channels rely on standardized organic values such as certification and pricing while short channels rely on product traceability, production methods, as well as the store/manager loyalty/reputation.

6.5.2. Distribution strategies to increase trust

The interviews aimed also at uncovering the distributors strategies used to increase trust towards organic food products and to address consumers' concerns. Results are presented by type of distribution channel in Table 2. It is clear that the common denominator to all distributors as well as certifiers and experts is consumers' education, "*If the government puts out some information, made it more available to the public, what organic actually meant, then that would increase the trust, and show people what it is supposed to achieve, and what it's not*". While almost all interviewees emphasize that education is a prerequisite to stabilize the demand and increase trust, this has to be nuanced. Consumer education can be seen from different angles: mass communication as part of a push strategy or providing information/building awareness as part of a pull strategy. These strategies are related to what has been said above regarding channel length. Hence, we can confidently associate pull strategies to short channels while push strategies are associated to long channels.

From a long channel perspective, retail chain managers suggest that price plays an important role in increasing consumers' trust. There is a lot of competition in the market and one way to differentiate the offering is to charge the lowest price to consumers; a price that reflects the organic value of what organic means to these consumers. One need to keep in mind that consumers shopping from these points of sale are not very knowledgeable about organics nor they buy organic for principle oriented reasons. According to the retail chain managers, their customers mainly buy organic for health reasons, but they also are price conscious.

Small grocery stores managers believe that trust should be increased if competition is to increase. The organic value marketed in this channel is mainly based on the relationship with the manager, the store reputation and also on the product/certification label. While pricing accuracy increases trust - if price reflects the value of OF products sold in these store - quality is not a key determinant to increase trust. Consumers associate quality with the store reputation and their relationship with the store manager, "*the consumer is trusting me as a store owner, if it says organic on my bins, and I am in turn trusting the company that I am buying it from*". It is important to note that all interviews have been conducted with independent storeowners. Hence, the involvement of the store managers/owner is more important than in retail chains. They unanimously state that consumers' education is key to increase loyalty and trust. They also argue that consumers are making smarter food choices but not all consumers are knowledgeable about organics. Hence, trust is increased by providing information about the product, the producer/farmer, and pricing.

As far as specialty stores go, the value offered in this channel is based on the width and depth of the product lines, and also on the traceability of organic foods via certification labels. Hence, education is crucial to keep current consumers and attract new ones. Education means information about the products and traceability. This is related – again – to the structure of the trust relationship. It is because of the type of store (specialty store) that expectations are different. Consumers expect that the quality is there and that the products are certified. This is also seen in the arguments put forward by the managers when asked about the reason why their customers buy organic; they mainly buy organic for heath, taste and environmental reasons. This is a clear indication that some of these consumers are very conscientious. Hence, the distribution strategies used to increase trust are mainly information driven; these are pull strategies.

Producers and farmers markets managers have the simplest distribution strategy. Most of these producers use direct channels and in most cases, they have small-scale operations. We have to keep in mind that most of these producers sell at farms gate and at the farmers market. They also supply some grocery stores or specialty stores. Hence, costs and margins are higher than in conventional channels. This is the only way to sustain the production operations as producers cannot offset the cost increase in their channel; i. e. , low sales volumes, keeping in mind that the organic value offered in these channels is based on the production methods. Hence, education is the key factor to increase trust, and of course the most important element is "knowing the producer". As stated previously, they focus their activity on building long-term relationship with their clientele to increase their market base. This offsets the price sensitivity effects. It is also important to note that there are two main types of producers, those who produce organic because of health and environmental reasons, and those who do it because of market reasons (profit driven). Hence, the perception of trust may differ depending on the size of the farm operations.

6.6. Sustainability

Distributors as well as experts discussed what they call *"industrial organic"*, *"conventional organic"*, and *"local organic"*. It is interesting to note that some distributors do not trust certification. Rather, they think that organic should be local and sustainable, especially when it comes to supporting the local economy and the farmers, *"I like supporting our local economy to that extent"*. Sustainability as a differentiation strategy as well as a trust enhancing strategy is not important in Canada yet. However, most distributors said that in the future, the organic food distribution system should factor in sustainability, as it may be a condition to access the market. One could draw the parallel with green products, as now recyclable packaging is the industry norm. Conversely, other distributors and experts were skeptical about sustainability and said that for now it does not add any value to the current market and it is not a differentiation strategy.

7. Discussion

This study attempts to provide readers with an overview of the structure and function of the market for organic food products in Canada based on the most current information available. In an attempt to produce a comprehensive picture, industry and government reports, academic papers, articles and personal communications have been reviewed for inclusion. Due to the difficulties inherent to the study of a relatively new market which includes players ranging from the private and not-for-profit to government and commercial/industrial, information on the Organic Food market remains partially incomplete. Further, to fill in the information gaps, a 2-prong design has been used along with a conceptual model of the existing organic processing and distribution structure. They are presented as a way to describe how the market has evolved. As can be seen in Figure 3 the production-market model takes into account the production/supply dynamics as well as the market dynamics.

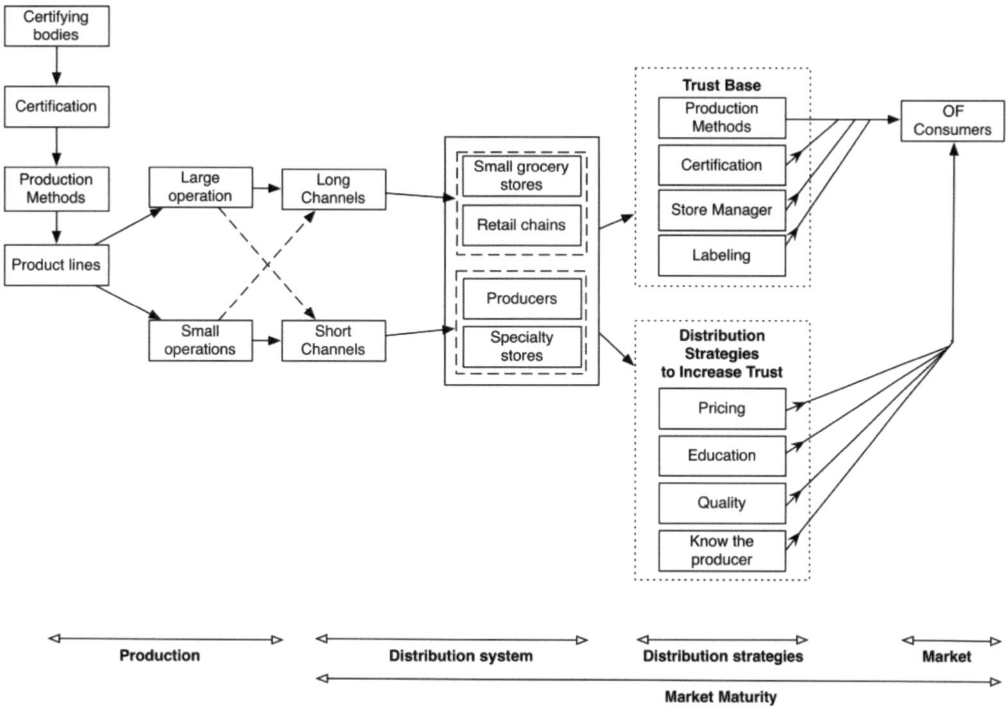

Figure 3. OF Market Model

Findings show that the organic market is the fastest growing sector in the food industry with double-digit market growth rates. Although organic agriculture is now going mainstream, demand remains concentrated in Europe and North America. However, these two regions are not self-sufficient because production is not meeting demand. It is also obvious that the supply is not located where the demand is. Hence, large volumes of organic imports, coming in from other regions, are used to balance the undersupply. The main problem for producers and growers is not with respect to demand for organic products but being able to supply that demand. Another issue with organic foods as with any food in the value chain is the multiple dimensions attached to organic products. Not only it is production based, but it is also distribution based. In fact, there is a clear differentiation between two distinct distribution perspectives: long channels versus short size channels. This shows the current divide in the organic food supply and demand. Long channels strategies are convenience and price driven. They offer an organic value targeted toward a certain consumer profile; these are customers that buy organic mainly for health reasons. Conversely, short channels are production method driven. These channels serve consumers having a principle-oriented life style; thus the environment and the support of the local economy are the main drives of this market demand along with health reasons; but price is not a concern. The organic market is also segregated by the entry of large commercial/industrial supply chains and the lack of existing small-scale infrastructure.

All players from the supply side also mention an increasing diversification of OF products and distribution channels. Further, it is clear that the OF industry is slowly integrating new product lines. These trends are directly dependent on the product life cycle [6]. In addition, the marketing of organic foods is not at maturity yet, leading to a lack of market standardization. Ultimately this discussion converges towards store choice and store positioning. Organic foods are value-based products, thus the OF purchasing framework is different than for conventional products. It is based on consumers trust orientations. Overall, distributors link consumers' trust in OF to different factors: organic labels, product labels, brands, traceability, advice, and/or store reputation. For consumers buying from supermarkets, organic labels are mainly what they trust, not brands. This is clearly different from results presented by [30] showing that OF consumers buying in supermarkets mainly rely on organic labels as well as brands. Consumers purchasing in specialty stores trust the store itself, the sales person advice, the products' traceability (transparency of the supply chain) and organic labels they know. Hence, communication on the products quality and traceability, advices and information provided by store managers and sales persons (and store reputation) could increase consumers' trust in OF. For consumers purchasing from producers and farmers markets, traceability is the main element of trust, which is addressed through a trustful relationship established between the producer and the consumer. Because of the differences in these trust dimensions and based on consumers' specific interests and knowledge, providing standard information for all OF consumers may not be the best communication strategy.

Suppliers provided also their perception on several organic consumers' characteristics that are in direct relation with the type of distribution channel used. For most suppliers, consumers are in general knowledgeable and are looking for authentic and healthy products, quality, and taste. Their level of knowledge as well as their motivation to consume organic products seems to differ depending on the point of sale they mostly use. In other words, consumers adopting short channels (producers/farmers market and specialty stores) are clearly looking for proximity with the producer, fresh products and quality, and a better understanding of the organic farming process. This segment shows a clear interest for the impacts of the production methods on health and on the environment. As mentioned by experts, there is a sub-segment in this target market that clearly differentiates between local food, industrial organic, and local organic. Conversely, consumers using standards channels of distribution – or long channels - are looking for convenience, healthy products and competitive prices. These consumers also seem to be confused between organic and natural products.

Lastly, certification and labeling systems serve as tools to enhance distribution and market development, create trust, and foster confidence. It is a commitment from producers/farmers to work with certain standards of production. According to [18], there are 80 countries using national standard of certification. Therefore, organic labels can be seen as an important source of trust. Several organic labels are now present on the Canadian market. This somehow induces some confusion, as some consumers do not know which one(s) to trust. Therefore, certification labels – assumed to play a central role - do not seem to have achieved that position in the OF consumers' decision-making process yet: they need to gain awareness, understanding and credibility in order to do so.

8. Conclusion

Consumers' interest in organic food has exhibited continued growth for the past two decades, which has attracted entrepreneurs and corporations seeing a big potential for this industry, and has also led to the creation of standards and regulations to guide the OF industry. Consumers are becoming more sophisticated in their purchasing decisions of OF, and companies are focusing on supply chain management in order to ensure high quality, traceability, and supply continuity. But the OF industry also faces some other challenges: (i) maintaining and increasing consumers' trust in the OF products and the OF industry in general, and (ii) facing new and fierce competition from market intermediaries and other types of "sustainable" products (e. g. fair trade products and local products). The OF industry and all its stakeholders will have to elaborate strategic responses to these opportunities and challenges that are in direct link with the supply level and the distribution structure. The results also provide an insight into the structure of the organic food industry and the determinants of consumers' trust. In fact, there are different levels of trust according to the channel members: trust related to the labeling and certification, trust related to the channel of distribution, and trust of the producer. These trust dimensions are direct consequences of the perceived added value to organic food provided by the producers, certifiers and distributors. This study has also some limitation, as results cannot be generalized. This research is exploratory and highlights the need to carry out quantitative and conclusive studies in order to generate not only conceptual clarifications but also answers regarding the Canadian organic food industry. This will in turn help to address implications of the consumer food consumption behavior for management and public policies.

Author details

Leila Hamzaoui-Essoussi and Mehdi Zahaf

Telfer School of Management, University of Ottawa, Canada

References

[1] Chryssohoidis, G. M. , Krystallis, A. Organic Consumers' Personal Value Research: Testing and Validating the List of Values (LOV) Scale Implementing A Value-Based Segmentation Task. Food Quality and Preference, 2005;16, 585-99.

[2] Torjusen, H. , Sandstad, L. , O'Doherty Jensen, K. , Kjaernes, U. European consumers' conceptions of organic food: A review of available research. Professional report 2004 (4).

[3] Knight, J. G. , Holdsworth, D. K. , Mather, D. W. Country-of-origin and choice of food imports: an in-depth study of European distribution channel gatekeepers. Journal of International Business Studies 2007; 38, 107-125.

[4] Urala, N. , Lahteenmaki, L. Reasons Behind Consumers' Functional Food Choice. Nutrition and Food Science 2003; 33 (4) 148-158.

[5] Canadian General Standards Board. Organic Production Systems General Principles and Management Standards,. Online Report CAN/CGSB-32; 2011, 310-2006.

[6] Hamzaoui-Essoussi, L. , Sirieix, L, Zahaf, M. What Would Make Consumers Trust Organic Products? A Qualitative Study Based on The Distributors' Perspective. Proceedings of the ECO-ENA: Economics & ECO-Engineering Associate, Ottawa, Canada, 2012; 33-52.

[7] Hall, A. , Veronika, M. Organic Farmers in Ontario: An Examination of the Conventionalization Argument. SociologiaRuralis 2001; 41 (4) 399-422.

[8] Jones, P. , Clarke-Hill, C. , Shears, P. , Hillier, D. Case Study: Retailing Organic Foods. British Food Journal 2001; 103 (5) 359-65.

[9] Tutunjian, J. Market Survey 2007. Canadian Grocer 2008; 122 (1) 26-34.

[10] Organic Monitor: The Global Market for Organic Food and Drink. Organic Monitor. London, 2007.

[11] Smithers, J. , Lamarche, J. , Alun, J. Unpacking the Terms of Engagement With Local Food at the Farmers' Market: Insights From Ontario. Journal of Rural Studies. 2008; 24 (3) 337-350.

[12] Rostoks, L. Romancing the Organic Crowd: this New Category May Yield Plenty Of Profits for You, if You Master the New Merchandising Rules to Attract the Organic Consumer. Canadian Grocer 2002; 116, 22-24.

[13] Eurostaf. ProduitsBio :Stratégies Comparées de la Grande Distribution en France. 2011.

[14] Tutunjian, J. Are Organic Products Going Mainstream?. Canadian Grocer 2004; 118, 31-34.

[15] AAFC, Agriculture and Agrifood Canada, 2008. Organic Production. http://www4. agr. gc. ca/AAFC AAC/display-afficher. do?id=1183748510661&lang=eng.

[16] Macey, A. Retail Sales of Certified Organic Food Products in Canada in 2006. Organic Agriculture Center of Canada, 2007http://www. organicagcentre. ca/Docs/RetailSalesOrganic_Canada2006. pdf

[17] Hamzaoui-Essoussi, L. , Zahaf, M. Exploring the Decision Making Process of Canadian Organic Food Consumers: Motivations and Trust Issues. Qualitative Market Research 2009; 12 (4) 443-459.

[18] Willer, H. , Kilcher, L. The World of Organic Agriculture. Statistics and Emerging Trends 2011. IFOAM, Bonn, &FiBL.

[19] Williams, P. R. D. , Hammitt, J. K. Perceived risks of conventional and organic produce: pesticides, pathogens and natural toxins. Risk Analysis 2001; 21 (92) 319-330.

[20] Baker, S. , Thompson, K. E. , Engelken, J. , Huntley, K. Mapping the values driving organic food choice: Germany vs t UK. European Journal of Marketing 2004; 38 (8) 995-1012.

[21] Chen, M. F. Attitude toward organic foods among Taiwanese as related to health consciousness, environmental attitudes, and the mediating effects of a healthy lifestyle. British Food Journal, 2009; 111 (2) 165-178.

[22] Makatouni, A. What motivates consumers to buy organic food in the UK? Results from a qualitative study. British Food Journal 2002; 104, 345-352.

[23] Fotopoulos, C. , Krystallis, A. , 2002. Purchasing motives and profile of the Greek organic consumer: a countrywide survey. British Food Journal 2002; (9) 730-764.

[24] Zanoli, R. ,Naspetti, S. Consumer motivations in the purchase of organic food: a means end approach. British Food Journal 2002; 104 (8) 643-653.

[25] Kihlberg, I. , Risvik, E. Consumers of organic foods – value segments and liking of bread. Food Quality and Preference 2007; 18 (3) 471-481.

[26] Padel, S. , Foster, C. Exploring the gap between attitudes and behavior – understanding why consumers buy or do not buy organic food. British Food Journal 2005; (8) 606-625.

[27] Verdurme, A. , Gellynck, X. , Viaene, J. Are organic food consumers opposed To GM food consumers. British Food Journal 2002; 104 (8) 610-623.

[28] Aertsens, J. , Verbeke, W. , Mondelaers, K. , Van Huylenbroeck, G. Personal determinants of organic food consumption: a review. British Food Journal 2009; 111 (10) 1140-1167.

[29] Kassarjian H. Content Analysis in Consumer Research. Journal of Consumer Research 1977; 4 (1) 8.

[30] Sirieix, L. , Pernin, SJ. -L. , Schaer, B. L'enjeu de la provenance régionale pour l'agriculture biologique. Innovations Agronomiques 2009; 4, 401-407.

Section 3

Alternative Feed

Chapter 8

The Use of Cactus as Forage for Dairy Cows in Semi-Arid Regions of Brazil

Marcelo de Andrade Ferreira, Safira Valença Bispo, Rubem Ramos Rocha Filho, Stela Antas Urbano and Cleber Thiago Ferreira Costa

Additional information is available at the end of the chapter

http://dx.doi.org/10.5772/53294

1. Introduction

The primary characteristic of semi-arid regions is frequent drought, which can be defined as a lack, scarcity, low frequency, and limited amount of rain or a poor distribution of rain during the winter period; therefore, a succession of drought years is not a rare occurrence in semi-arid regions[1]. Populations in these areas are predominantly rural, and the primary occupations of the workforce are in the agricultural sector. The combination of adverse environmental conditions and economic activity that is largely dependent on nature results in productive systems that are extremely vulnerable to unfavorable weather conditions.

Dairy farming has emerged as one of the few options in semi-arid regions, particularly in northeastern Brazil, where forage grown in pastures is the predominant source of feed for the herds. Native vegetation is used on a smaller scale and lends a number of seasonal attributes to the production in this region. According to [2], forage production largely occurs during the rainy season. Roughage supplementation, when used, consists of local fodder, such as prickly pear cactus, a crop that is widespread in the region, with or without concentrate supplements.

The spineless cactus is an important alternative for farmers due to its high productivity potential [2] and considerable survival and propagation capacity under conditions of little rain and high temperatures [3,4]. These properties have justified the use of the spineless cactus in this region to nearly 450 g/kg of the dry matter of the total diet. The spineless cactus can be successfully introduced into a diet due to its efficient water use [5]. According to [6], the spineless cactus is composed of 101 g/kg of dry matter (DM), 77 g/kg of crude protein (CP) and 278 g/kg of neutral detergent fiber (NDF).

In this context, cactus represents an extremely important feed source: it is well-adapted to the edaphic and climatic conditions of the region, and it is frequently used in dairy cattle feed, notably during periods of prolonged drought.

2. Chemical-bromatological composition of cactus

As shown in Table 1, the chemical-bromatological composition of cactus varies according to the species, age of the cladodes, and time of year [7].

Genus	DM (%)	CP[1]	NDF[1]	ADF[1]	TCH[1]	NFC[1]	MM[1]	Authors
Opuntia (Redonda)	10,40	4,20	--	--	--	--	--	[8]
Opuntia (gigante)	9,40	5,61	--	--	--	--	--	[7]
Opuntia (Redonda)	10,93	4,21	--	--	--	--	--	[7]
Nopalea (miúda)	16,56	2,55	--	--	--	--	--	[7]
Opuntia (gigante)	12,63	4,45	26,17	20,05	87,96	61,79	6,59	[9]
Opuntia (gigante)	8,72	5,14	35,09	23,88	86,02	50,93	7,98	[10]
Opuntia (gigante)	7,62	4,53	27,69	17,93	83,32	55,63	10,21	[11]
Nopalea (miúda)	13,08	3,34	16,60	13,66	87,77	71,17	7,00	[11]
Opuntia (gigante)	10,70	5,09	25,37	21,79	78,60	53,23	14,24	[12]
Opuntia (gigante)	14,40	6,40	28,10	17,60	77,10	--	14,60	[13]
Nopalea (miúda)	12,00	6,20	26,90	16,50	73,10	--	18,60	[13]
Opuntia (IPA-20)	13,80	6,00	28,40	19,40	75,10	--	17,10	[13]

[1]% at Dry Matter, DM = Dry Matter, CP = Crude Protein, NDF = Neutral Detergent Fiber, ADF = Acid Detergent Fiber, TCH = Total Carbohydrates, NFC = non-fibrous carbohydrates, MM = Mineral Matter.

Table 1. Chemical-bromatological composition of cactus

Regardless of the genus, cactus exhibits low levels of dry matter (DM, 11.69 ± 2.56%), crude protein (CP, 4.81 ± 1.16%), neutral detergent fiber (NDF, 26.79 ± 5.07%), and acid detergent fiber (ADF, 18.85 ± 3.17%). In contrast, cactus has high levels of total carbohydrates (TCH, 81.12 ± 5.9%), non-fibrous carbohydrates (NFC, 58.55 ± 8.13%), and mineral matter (12.04 ± 4.7%). The large amount of moisture found in the spineless cactus is in agreement with other reports [14,15]. This finding is very relevant to the arid and semi-arid regions in Northeastern Brazil, which suffer from a lack of available water for most of the year [16,17,18].

The crude protein in the spineless cactus varies depending on the species, the fertilization of the soil and the cultivation practices. The literature reports a low crude protein content for the spineless cactus. Due to this low protein content and the high content of non-fibrous carbohydrates, the spineless cactus is an excellent replacement for a portion of poor fodder. The cultivars most used are: **Palma gigante** (*Opuntia ficus-índica* – Mill), **Palma miúda** (*Nopalea cochenillifera* Salm-Dyck) and **Palma redonda** (*Opuntia ficus-índica* – Mill), where are illustrated in Figures 1, 2 and 3 respectively.

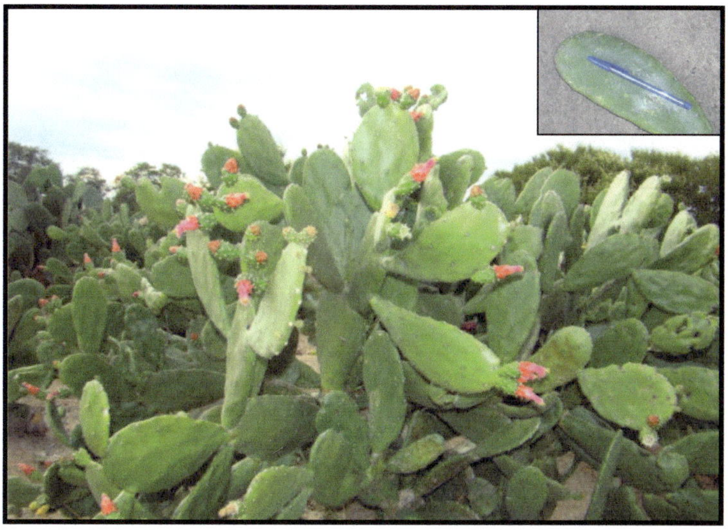

Figure 1. Palma Miúda – *Nopalea cochenillifera* Salm Dyck

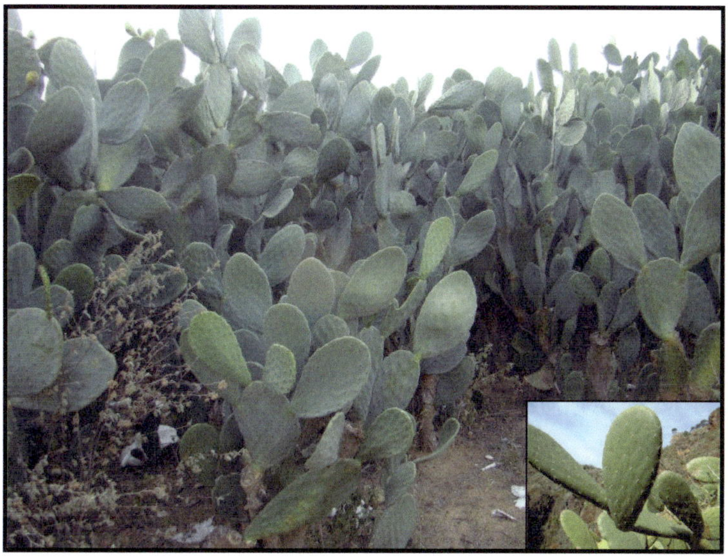

Figure 2. Palma Gigante – *Opuntia ficus-índica* Mill

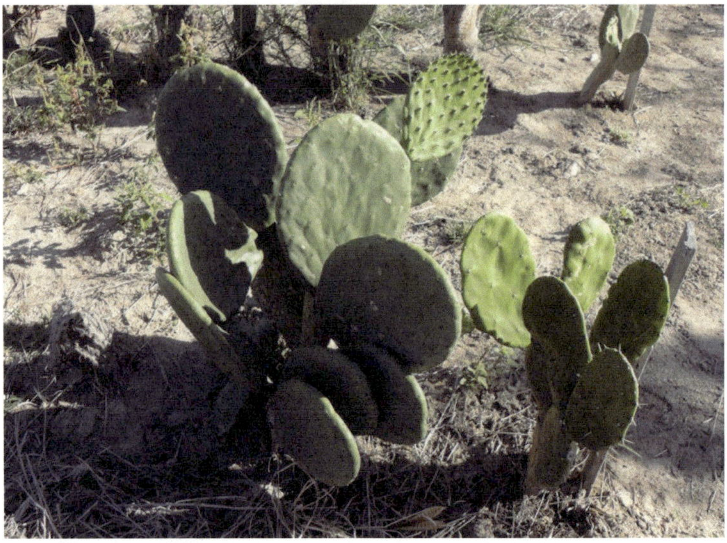

Figure 3. Palma Redonda – *Opuntia ficus-índica* - Mill

The high levels of calcium, potassium, and magnesium in cactus (Table 2) may reduce the absorption of these minerals, as well as limit microbial growth and the digestibility of different nutrients [19]. As with the majority of tropical forages, the amounts of phosphorous in cactus are considered low and insufficient for the needs of animals [20].

The calcium/phosphorus ratio ranged from 3.4: 1 to 22.5:1. [21] reported a calcium/phosphorus ratio that ranged from 8:1 to 11:3 and mean calcium and phosphorus contents ranging from 20 to 95 g/kg DM and 2.4 to 8.4 g/kg DM, respectively, depending on the age of the spineless cactus and the type of soil. However, in these studies, the phosphorus level was found to be 27 g/kg DM (Table 1); the lower value may possibly be due to the characteristics of the semi-arid soil in which the cactus was grown, where phosphorus levels are very low.

Genus	Minerals (% of DM)				Authors
	Ca	K	Mg	P	
Opuntia (gigante)	2.0	2.37	0.85	0.12	[22]
Opuntia (gigante)	2.35	2.58	-	0.16	[7]
Opuntia (gigante)	2.0	-	-	0.18	[23]
Opuntia (gigante)	2.87	-	-	0.36	[12]
Opuntia (gigante)	2.78	2.11	-	0.13	[24]
Opuntia (gigante)	4.1	-	1.3	0.5	[13]
Nopalea (miúda)	5.7	-	1.7	0.6	[13]
Nopalea (miúda)	2.25	1.5	-	0.1	[24]

Table 2. Mineral content of cactus

3. Energy content and digestibility of cactus

Measuring nutrient digestibility is the primary method for assessing the energy value of feeds. Using these values, the concentrations of digestible, metabolizable, and net energy can be estimated. There are also equations for estimating the energy value of feeds, such as those proposed by the [25], which estimate the total digestible nutrients (TDN) for maintenance by means of laboratory chemical analysis.

Table 3 lists the TDN content of cactus and other commonly used roughages in dairy cattle feed. The TDN content in cactus is higher than in any of the other roughages listed.

Feed	TDN[1] (% of DM)	$TDN_{NRC(2001)}$ (% of DM)	Authors
Cactus	64.33	65.91	[26]
Cactus	-	63.73	[12]
Cactus	-	61.13	[27]
Tifton hay	59.94	53.11	[26]
Sorghum silage	-	52.07	[12]
Corn silage	59.56	-	[28]
Elephant grass	49.59	-	[28]
Cane (1% urea)	60.57	-	[28]
Coastcross grass hay	50.24	-	[28]

[1]Estimated from a digestibility assessment

Table 3. Total digestible nutrient (TDN) content of various roughages

Digestion is defined as the process of converting macromolecules from food into simpler compounds that can be absorbed through the gastrointestinal tract [29]. A number of factors influence this process, such as the composition of the diet, any associative effects, the feed preparation and processing, the fodder maturity and the temperature of the surrounding environment, in addition to factors that are dependent upon the animals and their nutritional status, especially the energy density of the feed [30]. An excessive reduction in the fiber levels in the diet of ruminants can have a negative effect on the total digestibility of the feed. Fiber is fundamental to the maintenance of optimal conditions in the rumen because it alters the proportions of volatile fatty acids (VFAs), stimulates mastication and maintains the pH at adequate levels for microbial activity [31].

Cactus is a highly digestible roughage, with the round, giant, and small cultivars exhibiting *in vitro* DM digestibility coefficients of 74.4%, 75.0%, and 77.4%, respectively. The main difference between cactus and other forages is the degradability of the nutrients in the rumen [32]. The rumen degradability for several forages is listed in Table 4. These data indicate that among the forages studied, cactus has the largest water-soluble fraction, the highest rate of degradation for the fraction that is water-insoluble yet potentially degradable, and the greatest potential and effective degradabilities. [33] similarly observed higher *in vivo* and *in vitro* digestibility values for cactus compared to grass hay and alfalfa hay.

Table 4 lists the rumen degradability parameters of the DM, CP, and NDF observed for three varieties of cactus.

Item	Variety		
	Giant	Small	IPA-20
Dry matter (DM)			
a (g/kg of DM)	45	41	81
b (g/kg of DM)	908	872	882
kd (%/h)	7.5	8.1	7.3
ED[1] (g/kg of DM)	590	585	603
Crude protein (CP)			
a (g/kg of CP)	121	109	128
b (g/kg of CP)	884	891	872
kd (%/h)	6.0	5.9	6.2
ED[1] (g/kg of CP)	604	592	602
Neutral detergent fiber (NDF)			
a (g/kg of NDF)	56	49	50
b (g/kg of NDF)	668	703	698
Kd (%/h)	5.4	4.8	5.4
ED[1] (g/kg of NDF)	398	392	396

Adapted from [1]. [1] Considering a rate of passage of 5%/hour. a = water-soluble fraction; b = water-insoluble yet potentially degradable fraction; kd = rate of degradation of the b fraction

Table 4. Rumen degradation parameters (a, b, and kd) and effective degradability (ED) for three varieties of cactus

The data indicate that the different cactus components, particularly the DM, are highly degradable. Furthermore, the effective DM degradability values for the evaluated varieties of cactus are greater than those for other forages. This difference may be due to the high content of non-structural carbohydrates (NSC) found in cactus. High rumen degradability is associated with maximal rumen fermentation capacity and increases in the following: microbial protein synthesis, volatile fatty acid production, and nutrient absorption by the animal.

4. The use of cactus in the diet of dairy cattle

The regulation of the dry matter intake (DMI) is complex and is influenced by physical limitations and physiological and psychogenic factors. The physical factors include distention (a sensation of being full), the NDF concentration and the diet composition, which affect the digestion rate, the time elapsed for the reduction of particle size and the passage of the digested food. The physiological factors include the control of hunger and satiation by the hypothalamic region of the brain and psychogenic factors, which include herd behavior, feed palatability, environmental factors and stress [34]. Moreover, the [25] indicates a presumed negative correlation between the moisture and the DMI.

Cactus exhibits high palatability [35], and large quantities may be voluntarily consumed. Although cactus may be an excellent source of NFC (an important source of energy for ruminants), the low DM, NDF, and CP contents of cactus are insufficient for adequate animal performance.

Due to the low DM content of cactus, diets formulated with large proportions of cactus roughage typically have a high degree of moisture, which may be favorable in regions where water is scarce during certain seasons. [36] found that crossbred cows that produced approximately 15 kg of milk per day and received diets with 50% cactus drank almost no water. Similarly, [37] observed a complete lack of water consumption by dairy heifers fed diets with 64% cactus.

An adequate level of fiber is necessary in the diet of ruminants, particularly dairy cattle. Fiber is required for normal functioning of the rumen and associated activities, such as the following: rumination, ruminal motility, homogenization of the rumen content, salivary secretion (which helps stabilize the rumen pH in addition to providing more phosphorous for microbial fermentation), and maintenance of the correct content of milk fat [38]. The [25] has recommended that diets for lactating cows contain at least 25% NDF in the total DM and that 19% of the DM components be from roughage with high effectiveness. The NFC contents are between 36% and 44%, which reflects the NDF content in the diet and the proportion of NDF from roughage. Higher NFC values or lower NDF values may cause changes in the rumen fermentation pattern and a corresponding decrease in nutrient digestibility and milk fat content.

As indicated above, cactus has low NDF and high NFC contents, and these values should be taken into consideration when cactus is used in ruminant feed. Indiscriminate use of cactus as roughage has been found to cause several problems, including diarrhea, decreased milk fat content, reduced DM consumption, and weight loss, especially in lactating cows [8,39]. [6] previously emphasized the need to combine cactus with other roughages because cactus alone may increase the rate of passage through the digestive system and cause diarrhea.

In light of these observations, the combination of cactus with other roughages in dairy cattle diets was assessed (Table 5). Diarrhea, weight loss, changes in DM consumption, and reduced milk fat content were not observed. With regard to the feed composition, it should be noted that in all of the studies, the NDF and NFC contents were within the limit recommended by the [25] for maintaining normal rumen conditions. The authors provided evidence for the viability of low-cost feeds containing cactus and other roughages and demonstrated that milk production levels were similar to those obtained with more expensive feeds.

Roughage	MP	Cactus %	Roughage %	Concentrate %	NDF %	NFC %	Reference
SS	13.9	38.0	37.80	23.2	40.45	35.00	[23]
SB	13.6	55.4	17.80	25.3	36.00	39.00	
SS	29.5	29.00	28.00	43.00	34.00	41.50	[40]
TGH	17.6	49.81	25.35	22.31	34.60	42.39	[41]
EGH	17.6	46.66	27.98	22.33	33.91	42.26	
SB	16.2	50.05	24.07	22.34	36.38	41.47	
SS	25.7	24.00	33.00	43.00	31.90	43.42	[22]
SS	10.71	58.81	34.63	3.29	40.39	36.33	[42]
SuS	11.8	62.65	33.30	0.7	35.48	37.50	
GH	9.85	60.46	35.79	0.64	40.63	37.16	

Milk production (MP); sorghum silage (SS); sugarcane bagasse (SB); Tifton grass hay (TGH); elephant grass hay (EGH); sunflower silage (SuS); Guandu hay (GH)

Table 5. Combination of cactus with other roughages

When other roughages are combined with cactus, the balance between fibrous and non-fibrous carbohydrates in the diet should be considered alongside financial restrictions. The amount of cactus incorporated into diets rich in NDF and poor in NFC can be much greater than in diets with a greater level of concentrated feeds. All of these considerations can be summarized as a single objective: the elimination of such problems as diarrhea, low DM consumption, and weight loss, which are most often the result of an inefficient combination of feeds in cactus-based diets.

4.1. Cactus as a substitute for feed concentrate

The increasing cost of corn kernels reflects the following factors: its high value as a food product for human consumption, the need to use it in monogastric animal diets, and the demand for it in regions where it is not produced. The high NFC content of cactus has sparked interest in it as a substitute for energy concentrates and also in combination with non-protein nitrogen (NPN) sources, notably urea.

[43] substituted up to 75% of ground corn with cactus meal in a digestibility trial for cows and found no changes in the energy contents of the diets. It should be noted that consumption was restricted to 2.5% of the live weight of the animals. However, when cactus meal replaced 100% of the ground corn in the diets of growing sheep fed *ad libitum* [44], linear

reductions in the weight gain of the animals and in the TDN content of the diets were observed, although DM consumption was unaffected.

The total substitution of corn with fresh cactus and the partial substitution of soybean meal with fresh cactus and urea were studied in the diets of lactating cows (Table 6). An interesting finding of these studies was the minimal effect on milk production when corn was substituted with cactus in contrast to the changes in milk production that were observed when soybean meal was substituted with cactus. In general, reductions were observed in milk production when urea was included in the diets of lactating cows, regardless of the concentrate used with urea.

The most important observation was that the complete or partial substitution of concentrates with cactus lowered feed costs due to the reduced use of concentrates. Because there may be ways to compensate for the changes in milk production, this particular application of cactus is economically advantageous.

MPCF	Cactus %	Roughage %	*Corn %*	*Soybean %*	Urea %	NDF %	NFC %	CC kg	Reference
19.36	31.94	30.44	*14.27*	*21.95*	0.00	36.57	36.98	8.00	[12]
17.87	37.77	31.20	*13.92*	*14.04*	1.58	37.72	34.28	6.00	
15.90	36.00	37.00	*15.12*	*8.37*	1.89	39.64	36.68	3.70	[45]
14.83	50.00	37.00	*0.00*	*9.03*	1.69	39.80	33.28	1.30	
19.85	0.00	67.42	*16.39*	*14.19*	0.00	57.51	15.06	7.10	[46]
19.31	51.00	27.85	*0.00*	*19.15*	0.00	43.13	30.02	3.50	
13.66	45.00	30.00	*9.30*	*14.00*	0.20	40.00	34.70	4.40	[47]
11.12	60.00	30.00	*0.00*	*6.88*	1.63	41.50	34.40	1.30	

Milk production corrected for 4% fat (MPCF); concentrate consumption (CC)

Table 6. Cactus as a substitute for feed concentrate in the diets of lactating cows

4.2. Storage, preparation methods, and administration of the diet

In the majority of farms that use cactus as a feed resource for dairy cattle, the cactus is manually harvested and transported by horses, horse-drawn carts, or tractors. This typically occurs on a daily basis, which results in increased production costs. [48], studying the effects of different storage periods (0, 8, and 16 days) for giant cactus on dairy cattle performance, did not observe any effects on the composition of the cactus, DM consumption, and milk production by lactating cows in response to different storage periods. Similarly, there were no apparent losses in the DM and CP of cactus stored for up to 16 days [49]. These findings indicate that greater quantities of cactus can be harvested at a single time, regardless of whether it will be used immediately, to minimize costs associated with harvest and transportation.

The most common approach to administering cactus to dairy cattle is mincing it in the trough without mixing it with any other roughage. The concentrate, when used, should be offered at the time of milking. When the feeds are supplied separately in this manner, it is not always possible to obtain an accurate estimate of the real intake of these feeds, especially when more than one type of roughage is consumed. This difficulty in measuring is due to a preference for certain feeds, making it difficult to calculate the average individual consumption and to characterize the diet ingested by the animal. It is important to stress that roughage rich in NFC, such as cactus, may cause a number of rumen disorders when provided separately and in large amounts. As a result, the use of the complete ration or TMR (total mixed ration) has become a common practice for regulating the composition of the diet [29]. These approaches also contribute to the supply of the diet, which should provide an adequate balance of nutrients. As a result, the use of the complete ration or TMR (Figure 4) has become a common practice for regulating the composition of the diet.

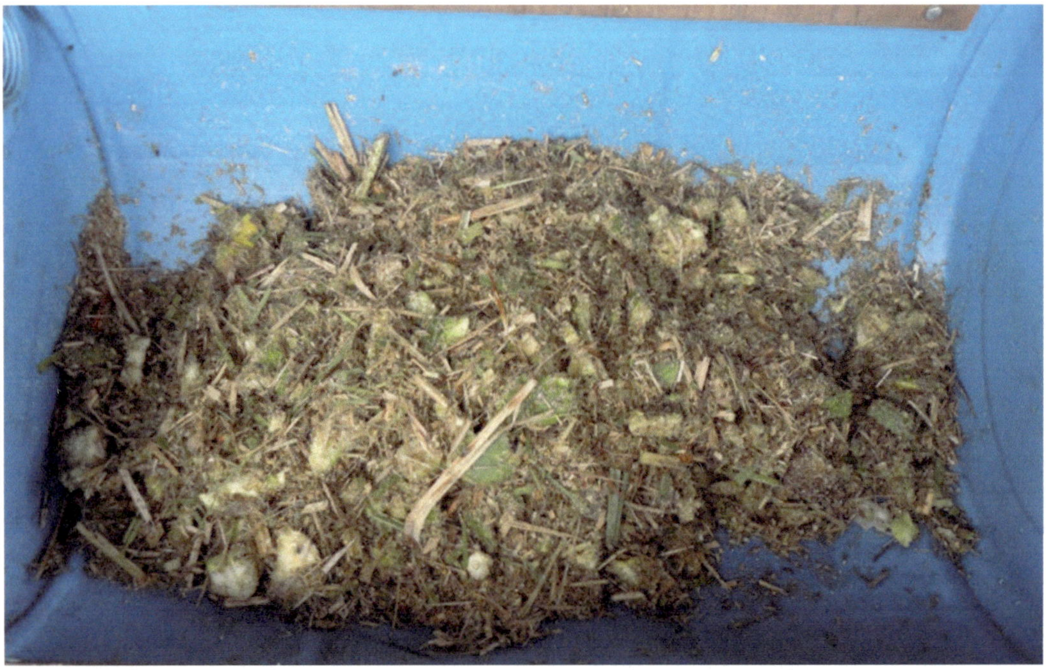

Figure 4. Total mixed ration containing spineless cactus

[50] previously reported that diets consisting of cactus, sorghum silage, and concentrate should be provided in the form of a complete mixture (Table 8).

The authors observed that the proportion of ingredients in the diet actually consumed was different than that of the diet offered, especially when the ingredients were provided separately. In such cases, animals consumed smaller amounts of sorghum silage, which led to a reduced amount of effective fiber along with a decrease in rumination and chewing.

Changes in the amount of milk fat indicated that the production of saliva was probably also decreased, which would have subsequent effects on rumen conditions [51]. The NDF and NFC contents in the diet were 30.3% and 39.22%, respectively. These values are notably close to the limits recommended by the [25] for maintaining rumen health and milk fat. Thus, any changes in the proportion of feed components could significantly alter these values and the nutritional balance of the feed supplied to the animals. According to [52], the balance of structural and non-structural carbohydrates is important for animal health and function along with nutrient utilization, which is one of the intended goals of providing the diet as a complete mixture. A better utilization of energy for milk production was also observed when using a complete mixture feeding strategy, rather than supplying the ingredients separately [53]. A better utilization of energy for milk production was also observed when using a complete mixture feeding strategy, rather than supplying the ingredients separately (Figure 5)

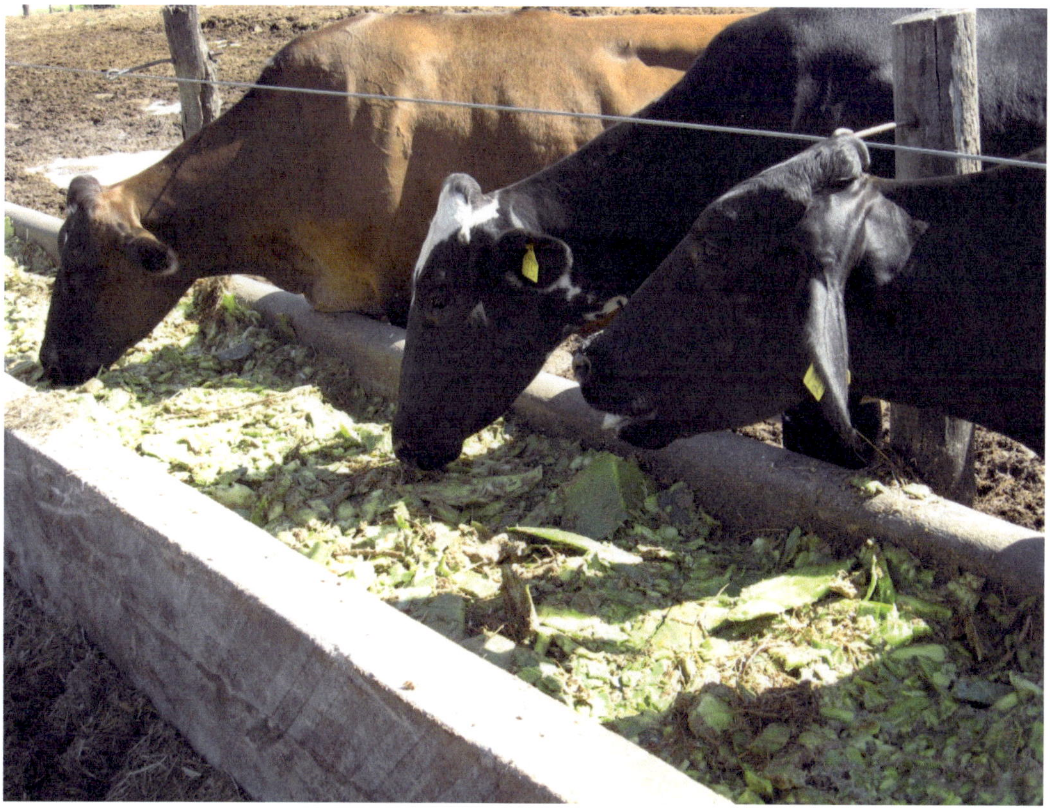

Figure 5. Dairy cows eating total mixed ration.

In addition to the supply strategy, another aspect that warrants attention is the way in which the cactus is processed (Figure 6, 7, 8 and 9). Generally, the cactus is minced with a knife or with specific forage equipment. The difference between the two types of processing is that mincing with a knife does not lead to mucilage exposure, while the use of forage equipment does. When cactus was combined with sugarcane bagasse and soybean meal and fed to lactating cows, higher consumption rates were observed when the cactus was passed through a forage machine compared to processing with a knife (16.3 versus 15.2 kg/day, respectively) [54]. This result probably reflects the exposure of the mucilage, which adheres to the other feed components. As a result, feed selectivity is reduced, and consumption of the complete feed, including unpalatable components such as sugarcane bagasse, is facilitated. Animals that received cactus minced with a knife had a greater opportunity to select particular feed components, which resulted in an imbalance of structural and non-structural carbohydrates in the diet. In turn, this imbalance led to a reduction in milk fat compared to animals fed cactus processed using a forage machine (36 versus 39 g/kg, respectively).

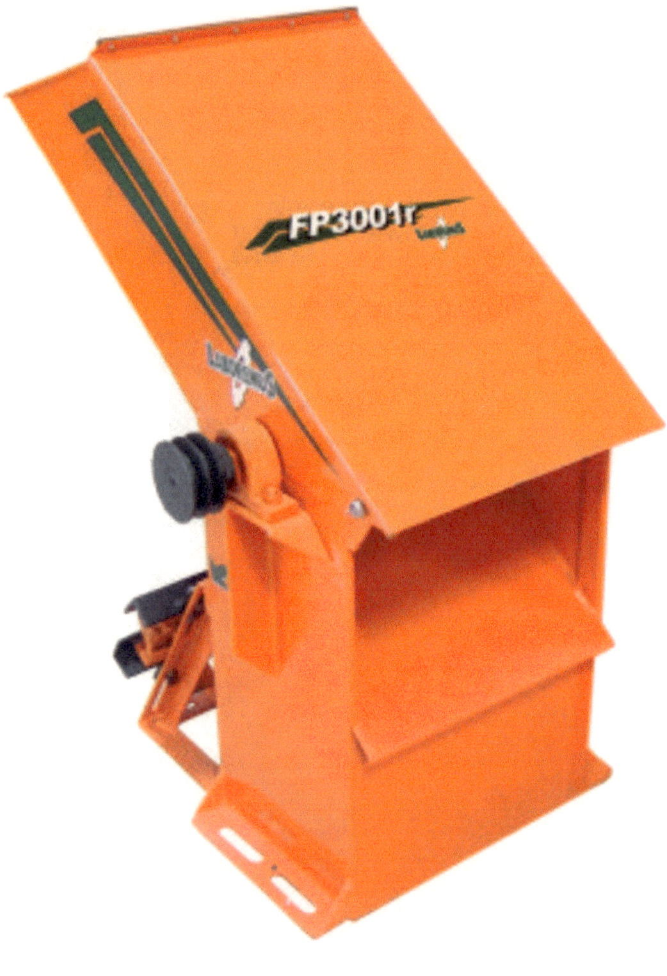

Figure 6. Forage machine

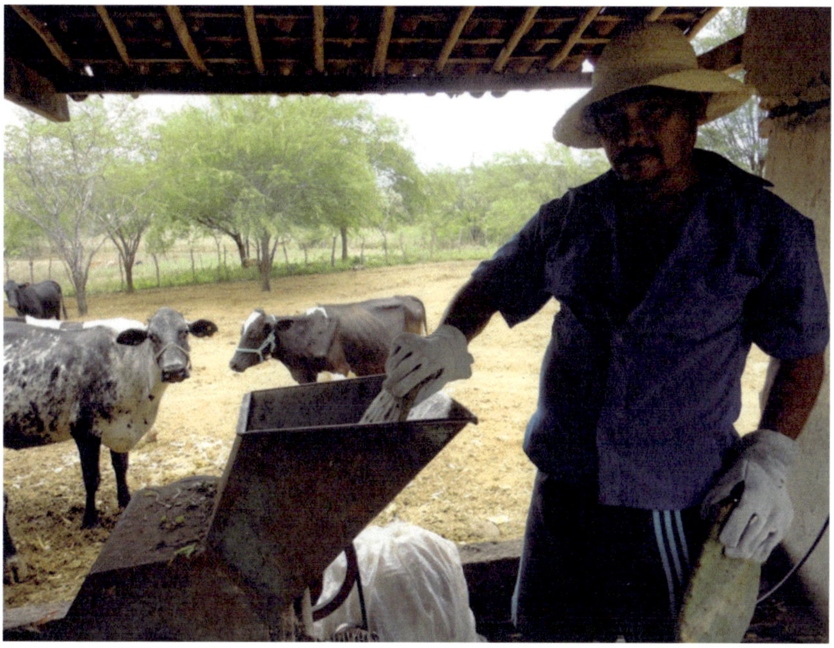

Figure 7. The laborer doing the process

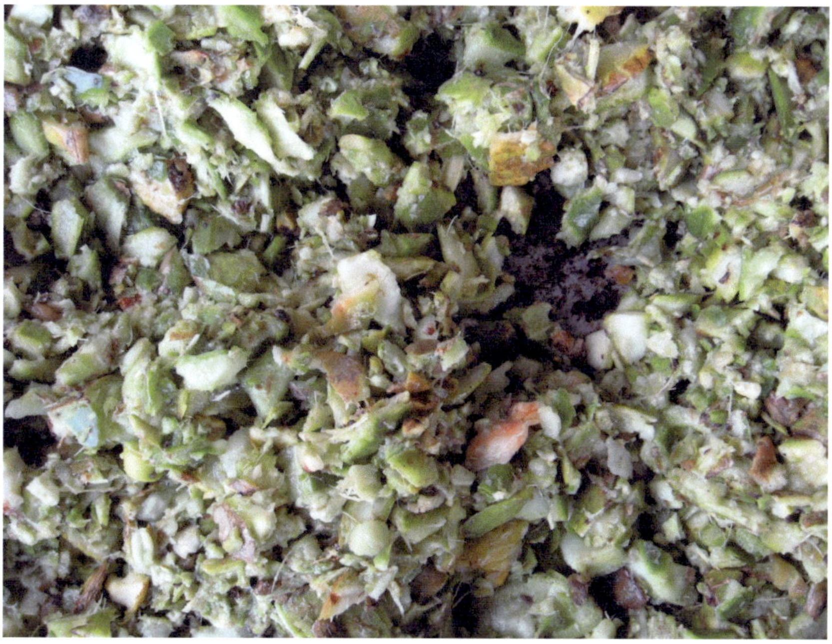

Figure 8. Spineless cactus processed in machine

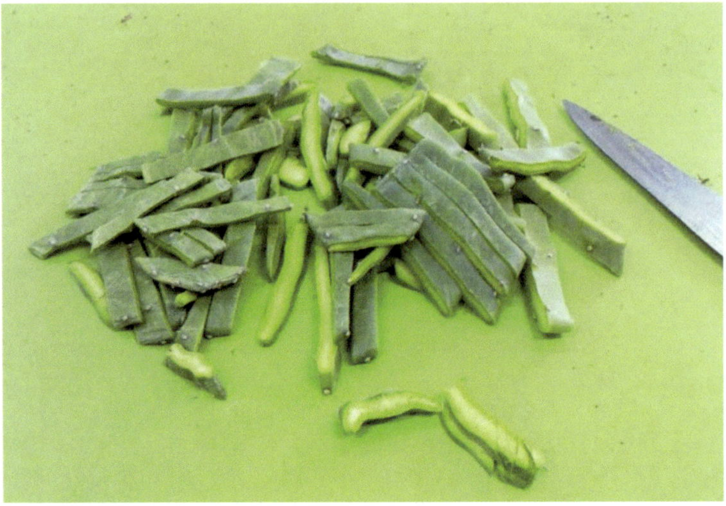

Figure 9. Spineless cactus minced with a knife

4.3. Cactus in the diet of heifers

The establishment of an efficient rearing system, mainly of females, is a challenge for the majority of milk producers. Although heifers should receive appropriate feed and management to reach an ideal weight for breeding and to start productive life earlier, there are important economic considerations. It is therefore necessary to strike a balance between calving at an early age and economic factors. The feeding plan adopted for the heifers should allow for the weight at puberty and first mating to be reached as soon and economically as possible. In semi-arid regions, achieving this goal requires supplementation of the diets with roughage and concentrate feeds.

The literature on the use of cactus in the diets of growing dairy cattle is limited; a portion of the available data is listed in Table 7.

Breed	Cactus %	Bagasse %	Urea %	Supplement (kg/day)	WG (kg/day)	Reference
Holstein	69.80	27.60	2.60	Wheat meal (1)	0.71	[55]
Holstein	69.80	27.60	2.60	Soybean meal (1)	1.20	
Crossbred*	64.00	30.00	4.00	Wheat meal (1)	0.60	[37]
Crossbred*	64.00	30.00	4.00	Soybean meal (1)	0.72	
Crossbred*	64.00	30.00	4.00	Cotton meal (1)	0.84	
Crossbred*	64.01	30.01	4.01	Cottonseed (1)	0.75	
Crossbred*	64.02	30.02	4.02	No supplement	0.43	

*5/8 Holstein/Gir

Table 7. Cactus in the diets of growing heifers

http://dx.doi.org/10.5772/53294

5. Spineless cactus in organic farming and food production

Brazil has the second largest area of organic farming in the world, being second only to Australia. The country holds the largest consumer market for organic foods in South America since the data is based on survey means that was conducting between January and February this year by the Coordination of Agroecology of the Ministry of Agriculture, Livestock and Supply – MAPA.

Organic agriculture presents as a cost-effective and relevant alternative to small farmers which it can also be an important way to people from countryside and downtown have health food easily. The aim is to produce healthy vegetables, grains and meat, providing ecological balance at the ground without harming the environment. As a social view that combination can increase the life quality of countryside's families, the value of the local cultural and it can supply the livelihood to farmers too.

The spineless cactus has being great potential in organic animal production system where it has traditionally been grown with the use of organic manure, especially because manure is considerably to increases the green matter per hectare, figure 10. As an example, considering a production of 175 tons of green matter (GM) per hectare per year, and a cow consuming 60 kg per day of spineless cactus, that production might be enough to feed 12 cows per hectare for about 240 days.

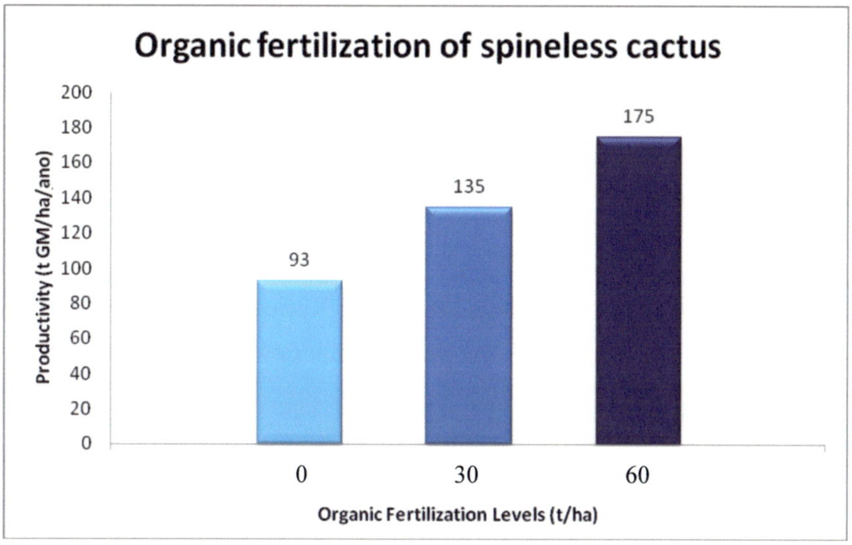

Figure 10. Effect of organic fertilization in the production of spineless cactus Source: [56]

In the semiarid region of Brazilian there is already success stories about the example cited above, as Timbaúba Farm Organic Food Ltd. - Cacimbinhas / AL. The Farm is about a thousand hectares of land operates a livestock complex integrated with nature, where it takes almost all the inputs needed to produce. The property was one of the pioneers of the country, and it was the fourth company to receive certification seal advice given by IBD in 2002.On that farm the spineless cactus is one of the feeds produced to supply for herd.

6. Conclusion

The spineless cactus is presented as a forage crop vital to the sustainability of farming systems in semi-arid regions, primarily as an energy source. Information about your use rationally in ruminant diets has been obtained, and therefore must be effectively adopted. Aspects such as providing complete diet and association with bulky and nitrogen sources, are basic premises when the use of spineless cactus. As seen, it is possible to provide it in large quantities to ruminants, regardless of the animal category, the physiological stage and the purpose of the production system.

The combination of cactus and urea represents a viable option because it provides adequate energy and sufficient nitrogen for the microorganisms in the rumen. The high concentration of soluble carbohydrates in cactus facilitates the incorporation of nitrogen into microbial protein, which is the main source of metabolizable protein for the host animal. In this manner, the protein content of cactus, which is normally insufficient for adequate animal performance, may be increased. Furthermore, combining cactus with sugarcane bagasse, which has a high NDF content (of low nutritional value), makes it possible to improve nutrient absorption because sugarcane bagasse introduces effective fiber into the system. The increased fiber promotes rumen health and improves the absorption of nutrients from the diet. In addition to the cactus-fiber-NPN triad, providing a supplementary source of amino acids (true protein) is also an important consideration.

Acknowledgements

The Federal Rural University of Pernambuco which provided the facilities and animals to perform this experiments. The authors would also like to thank CNPq (National Council for Scientific and Technological Development) for funding the researchs.

Author details

Marcelo de Andrade Ferreira[1], Safira Valença Bispo[2], Rubem Ramos Rocha Filho[1], Stela Antas Urbano[1] and Cleber Thiago Ferreira Costa[1]

*Address all correspondence to: ferreira@dz.ufrpe.br

1 University Federal Rural of Pernambuco / Animal Science, Brasil

2 University Federal of Paraiba / Animal Science, Brasil

References

[1] Ferreira, MA. Palma Forrageira na Alimentação de Bovinos Leiteiros. Recife: Universidade Federal Rural de Pernambuco; 2005.

[2] Dubeux Jr JCB, Santos MVF, Lira MA, Santos DC, Farias I, Lima LE, Ferreira RLC. Productivity of Opuntia ficus-indica (L.) Miller under Different N and P Fertilization and Plant Population in North-East Brazil. Journal of Arids Environments 2006; 67(3) 357–372.

[3] Nobel, PS Ecophysiology of Opuntia ficus-indica. In: Mondragón-Jacobo, C; Pérez-González, S. (Eds.) Cactus (Opuntia spp.) as forage. Rome: Food and Agriculture Organization of the United Nations, 2001. p.13-20.

[4] Reynolds, S.G.; Arias, E. Introduction. In: Mondragón-Jacobo, C.; Pérez-González, S. (Eds.). Cactus (Opuntia spp.) as forage. Rome: Food and Agriculture Organization of the United Nations, 2001. p.1-4.

[5] Snyman, H.A. A case study on in situ rooting profiles and water-use efficiency of cactus pears, Opuntia ficus-indica and Opuntia robusta. 2005. Available in http://www.jpacd.org/v7/v7p1-215snymo.pdf.

[6] Ben Salem H, Nefzaoui A, Ben Salem L. Supplementing Spineless Cactus (Opuntia ficus-indica f. inermis) Based Diets with Urea-Treated Straw or Oldman Saltbush (Atriplex nummularia). Effects on Intake, Digestion and Sheep Growth. Journal of Agricultural Science 2002; 138(1) 85–92.

[7] Santos MVF. Composição Química, Armazenamento e Avaliação da Palma Forrageira (Opuntia ficus indica Mill. e Nopalea cochenillifera Salm Dyck) na Produção de leite. M.Sc. thesis. Universidade Federal Rural de Pernambuco; 1989.

[8] Santana OP, Viana SP, Estima AL, Farias I. Palma versus Silagem na Alimentação de Vacas Leiteiras. Revista Brasileira de Zootecnia 1972; 1(1) 31-40.

[9] Andrade DKB, Ferreira MA, Véras ASC, Wanderley WL, Silva LE, Carvalho FFR, Alves KS, Melo WS. Apparent Digestibility and Absorption of Holstein Cows Fed Diets with Forage Cactus (Opuntia fícus-indica Mill) in Replacement of Sorghum Silage (Sorghum bicolor (L.) Moench). Revista Brasileira de Zootecnia 2002; 31(5) 2088-2097.

[10] Magalhães MCS, Véras ASC, Carvalho FFR, Ferreira MA, Melo JN, Melo WS, Pereira JT, Lira MA. Inclusion of Broiler Litter in Forage Cactus Based Diets (Opuntia ficus-indica Mill) for Lactating Crossbred Cows. 2. Apparent Digestibility. Revista Brasileira de Zootecnia 2004; 33(6) 1909-1919.

[11] Araújo PRB. Substituição do Milho por Palma Forrageira (Opuntia ficus-indica Mill. e Nopalea cochenillifera Salm-Dyck) em Dietas Completas para Vacas em Lactação. M.Sc. thesis. Universidade Federal Rural de Pernambuco; 2002.

[12] Melo AAS, Ferreira MA, Véras ASC, Lira MA, Lima, LE, Vilela MS, Melo, EOS, Araújo PRB. Partial Replacement of Soybean Meal for Urea and Forage Cactus in Lactating Cows Diets. I. Performance. Revista Brasileira de Zootecnia 2003; 32(3) 727-736.

[13] Batista AM, Mustafa AF, McAllister T, Wang Y, Soita H, Mckinnon JJ. Effects of Variety on Chemical Composition, In Situ Nutrient Disappearance and In Vitro Gas Production of Spineless Cacti. Journal of the Science of Food and Agriculture 2003; 83(5), 440-445.

[14] Alary, V., Nefzaoui, A., & Ben Jemaa, M. Promoting the adoption of natural resource management technology in arid and semi-arid areas: Modelling the impact of spineless cactus in alley cropping in Central Tunisia. Agricultural Systems 2007, 94(2), 573–585.

[15] Gebremariam, T.; Melaku, S.; Yami, A. Effect of wilting of cactus pear (Opuntia ficus-indica) on feed utilization in sheep. Tropical Science 2006,46(1) 37-40.

[16] Ben Salem H, Nefzaoui A, Ben Salem L. Spineless cactus (Opuntia ficus-indica f. inermis) and oldman saltbush (Atriplex nummularia L.) as alternative supplements for growing Barbarine lambs given straw-based diets. Small Ruminant Research. 2004;51(1) 65–73.

[17] Bispo, SV.; Ferreira, MA.; Véras, ASC.; Batista, AMV.; Pessoa, RAS.; Bleuel, MP. Palma forrageira em substituição ao feno de capim-elefante. Efeito sobre consumo, digestibilidade e características de fermentação ruminal em ovinos. Revista Brasileira de Zootecnia 2007, 36(6) 1902-1909.

[18] Sirohi SK, Karmis SA, Misra AK. Nutrient intake and utilization in sheep fed with prickly pear cactus. Arid Environ 1997; 36 161–166.

[19] Ben Salem H, Nefzaoui A, Abdouli H, Orskov ER. Effect of Increasing Level of Spineless Cactus (Opuntia ficus indica var. inermes) on Intake and Digestion by Sheep Given Straw Based Diets. Animal Science 1996; 62(1) 293-299.

[20] Germano RH, Barbosa HP, Costa, RG et al. Avaliação da Composição Química e Mineral de Seis Cactáceas do Semi-Árido Paraibano. In: anais da 28ª reunião anual da Sociedade Brasileira de Zootecnia, 1991, João Pessoa, Brasil.

[21] Mondragon-Jacobo, C., and S. Perez-Gonzalez. Cactus (Opuntia spp) as forage. FAO Plant Production and Protection Paper 169. FAO, Rome, Italy; 2001.

[22] Wanderley WL, Ferreira MA, Andrade DKB, Véras ASC, Farias I, Lima EL, Dias AMA. Replacement of Forage Cactus (Opuntia ficus indica Mill) for Sorghum Silage (Sorghum bicolor (L.) Moench) in the Dairy Cows Feeding. Revista Brasileira de Zootecnia 2002; 31(1) 273-281.

[23] Mattos LME, Ferreira MA, Santos DC, Lira MA, Santos MVF, Batista AMV, Véras, ASC. Association of Forage Cactus (Opuntia ficus indica Mill) with Different Fiber Sources on Feeding of Crossbreed 5/8 Holstein-Zebu Lactating Cows. Revista Brasileira de Zootecnia 2000; 29(6) 2128-2134.

[24] Santos MVF, Lira MA, Farias I. Estudo Comparativo das Cultivares de Palma Forrageira Gigante, Redonda (Opuntia ficus indica Mill.) e Miúda (Nopalea cochenillifera Salm-Dyck) na Produção de Leite. Revista Brasileira de Zootecnia 1997; 19(6) 504-511.

[25] National Research Council - NRC. Nutrient Requirements of Dairy Cattle. Washington: D.C.; 2001.

[26] Mendes Neto J. et al. Determinação do NDT da Palma Forrageira (Opuntia fícus indica Mill. cv. Gigante). In: anais da 40ª reunião anual da Sociedade Brasileira de Zootecnia, 2003, Santa Maria, Brasil.

[27] Magalhães, M.C.S. Cama de frango associada à palma forrageira (Opuntia ficus-indica Mill) na alimentação de vacas mestiças em lactação. Recife: Universidade Federal Rural de Pernambuco, 2002. 73p. Dissertação (Mestrado em Zootecnia) - Universidade Federal Rural de Pernambuco, 2002.

[28] Rocha Júnior VR, Valadares Filho SC, Borges AM, Magalhães KA, Ferreira CCB, Valadares RFD, Paulino MF. Determination of Energy Value of Feed for Ruminants by Equation Systems. Revista Brasileira de Zootecnia 2003; 32(2) 473-479.

[29] Van Soest, PJ. Nutritional Ecology of the Ruminant (2nd Ed.). Cornell University Press, Ithaca: New York; 1994.

[30] Church, D.C. Gusto, apetito e regulacion de la ingesta de alimentos; In: Church, D. C. (Ed.) Fisiologia digestiva y nutricion de los ruminantes. Zaragoza: Acribia, 1974. p. 405-435.

[31] MERTENS, D.R. Análise da fibra e sua utilização na avaliação de alimentos e formulação de rações: In: 29ª Reunião Anual da Sociedade Brasileira de Zootecnia, 1992, Lavras, Brasil. Anais. Lavras, Brasil: 1992, p.188-219.

[32] Nefzaoui A, Ben Salem H. Opuntia spp. A Strategic Fodder and Efficient Tool to Combat Desertification in the WANA Region. In: Mondragon-Jacobo C, Perez-Gonzalez S. (ed.) Cactus (Opuntia spp.) as Forage. Rome: FAO; 2001. p73–90.

[33] Shoop MC, Alford EJ, Mayland HF. Plains Pricklypear is a Good Forage for Cattle. Journal of Range Management 1977; 30(1) 12-16.

[34] Doughterty, C.T.; Collins, M. Forage utilization. In: Barnes, R.F.; Miller, D.A.; Nelson, C.J. (Eds).Forages: an introduction to grassland agriculture forages an introduction to glassland agriculture. 6.ed. Ames: Iowa State University Press, 2003. p.391-414.

[35] Tegegne F, Kijora C, Peters KJ. Study on the Effects of Incorporating Various Levels of Cactus Pear (Opuntia ficus-indica) on the Performance of Sheep. In:Tielkes E, Hulsebusch C, Hauser I, Deininger A, Becker C. (eds.) The Global Food & Product Chain – Dynamics, Innovation, Conflicts, Strategies: proceedings of the Conference on International Agricultural Research for development, 11-13 october 2005, Stuttgart, Germany.

[36] Lima RMB, Ferreira MA, Brasil LHA, Araújo PRB, Véras ASC, Santos DC, Cruz Maom, Melo AAS, Oliveira TN, Souza IS. Replacement of the Corn by Forage Cactus:

Ingestive Behavior of Crossbreed Lactating Cows. Acta Scientiarum. Animal Sciences 2002; 25(2) 347-353.

[37] Pessoa RAS. Forage Cactus, Sugar Cane Bagasse and Urea for Heifers and Lactating Cows. M.Sc. thesis. Universidade Federal Rural de Pernambuco; 2007.

[38] Mertens DR. Creating a System for Meeting the Fiber Requeriments of Dairy Cows. Journal of Dairy Science 1997; 80(7) 1463-1481.

[39] Santos, M.V.F., Lira, M.A., Farias, I. et al.. Estudo comparativo das cultivares de palma forrageira gigante redonda (Opuntia ficus indica Mill.) e miúda (Nopalea cochenillifera Salm-Dyck.) na produção de leite. Revista Brasileira de Zootecnia 1990, 19(6):504-511.

[40] Melo AAS, Ferreira MA, Véras ASC, Lira MA, Lima LE, Pessoa RAS, Bispo SV, Cabral AMB, Azevedo M. Dairy Cows Performance Fed Whole Cottonseed in a Forage of Cactus-Base Diet. Acta Scientiarum. Animal Sciences 2006; 41(7) 1165-1171.

[41] Silva RR, Ferreira MA, Véras ASC, Ramos AO, Melo AAS, Guimarães AV. Addition of Spineless Cactus (Opuntia ficus indica Mill) to Different Types of Roughage in the Diet of Lactating Holstein Cows. Acta Scientiarum. Animal Sciences 2007; 29(3) 317-324.

[42] Wanderley WL. Silagens e Fenos em Associação à Palma Forrageira para Vacas em Lactação e Ovinos. M.Sc. thesis. Universidade Federal Rural de Pernambuco; 2008.

[43] Véras RML, Ferreira MA, Carvalho FFR, Véras ASC. Forage Cactus (Opuntia ficus-indica Mill) Meal in Replacement of Corn. 1. Apparent Digestibility of Nutrients. Revista Brasileira de Zootecnia 2002; 31(3) 1302-1306.

[44] Véras RML, Ferreira MA, Cavalcanti CVA, Véras ASC, Carvalho FFR, Santos GRA, Alves KS, Maior Junior RJS. Replacement of Corn by Forage Cactus Meal in Growing Lambs Diets. Performance. Revista Brasileira de Zootecnia 2005; 34(1) 249-256.

[45] Araújo PRB, Ferreira MA, Brasil LHA, Santos DC, Lima RB, Véras ASC, Santos MVF, Bispo SV, Azevedo M. Replacement of Corn by Forage Cactus in the Total Mixed Rations for Crossbreed Lactating Cows. Revista Brasileira de Zootecnia 2004; 33(6) 1850-1857.

[46] Oliveira VS, Ferreira MA, Guim A, Modesto EC, Lima LE, Silva FM. Total Replacement of Corn and Partial of Tifton Hay by Forage Cactus in Diets for Lactating Dairy Cows. Intake and Digestibility. Revista Brasileira de Zootecnia 2007; 36(5) 1419-1425.

[47] Bispo SV. Substituição Total do Milho e Parcial do Farelo de Soja por Palma Forrageira e Uréia para Vacas em Lactação. D.Sc. thesis. Universidade Federal Rural de Pernambuco; 2009.

[48] Santos MVF, Farias I, Lira MA, Nascimento MMA, Santos DC, Tavares Filho JJ. Storage Time of Forage Cactus (Opuntia ficus indica Mill) on the Performance of Lactating Dairy Cows. Revista Brasileira de Zootecnia 1998; 27(1) 33-39.

[49] Santos MVF, Lira MA, Farias I. et al. Efeito do período de armazenamento pós-Colheita sobre o Teor de Matéria Seca e Composição Química das Palmas Forrageiras. Pesquisa Agropecuária Brasileira 1992; 27(6) 777-73.

[50] Pessoa RAS, Ferreira MA, Lima LE, Lira MA, Véras ASC, Silva AEVN, Sosa MY, Azevedo M, Miranda KF, Silva FM, Melo AAS, López ORM. Respuesta de Vacas Lecheras Sometidas a Diferentes Estratégias de Alimentación. Archivos de Zootecnia 2004; 53(203) 309-320.

[51] Allen MS. Relationship between Fermentation Acid Productions in the Rumen the Requirement for Physically Effective Fiber. Journal of Dairy Science 1997; 80(7) 1447-1462.

[52] Nocek, JE, Russel JB. Protein and Energy as an Integrated Systems. Relationship of Ruminal Protein and Carbohydrate Avaliability to Microbial Synthesis and Milk Production. Journal of Dairy Science 1988; 71(8) 2070-2107.

[53] Yrjänen S, Kaustell K., Kangasniemi, R., Sariola, J., Khalili, H. Effects of Concentrate Feeding Strategy on the Performance of Dairy Cows Housed in a Free Stall Barn. Livestok Production Science 2003; 81(2) 73-81.

[54] Vilela MS, Ferreira, MA, Azevedo M, Modesto EC, Farias I, Guimarães AV, Bispo SV. Effect of Processing and Feeding Strategy of the Spineless Cactus for Lactating Cows: Ingestive Behavior. Applied Animal Behavior Science 2010; 125(1) 1-8.

[55] Carvalho MC, Ferreira MA, Cavalcanti CVA, Lima LE, Silva FM, Miranda KF, Véras ASC, Azevedo M, Vieira VCF. Association of Sugar Cane Bagasse, Forage Cactus and Urea with Different Supplements in Diets of Holstein Heifers. Acta Scientiarum. Animal Sciences 2005; 27(2) 247-252.

[56] Gomes JB. Adubação orgânica na produção de palma forrageira (Opuntia fícus índica – Mill) no cariri paraibano. M.Sc. thesis. Universidade Federal de Campina Grande; 2011.